Early Career Physician Mental Health and Wellness

W0228155

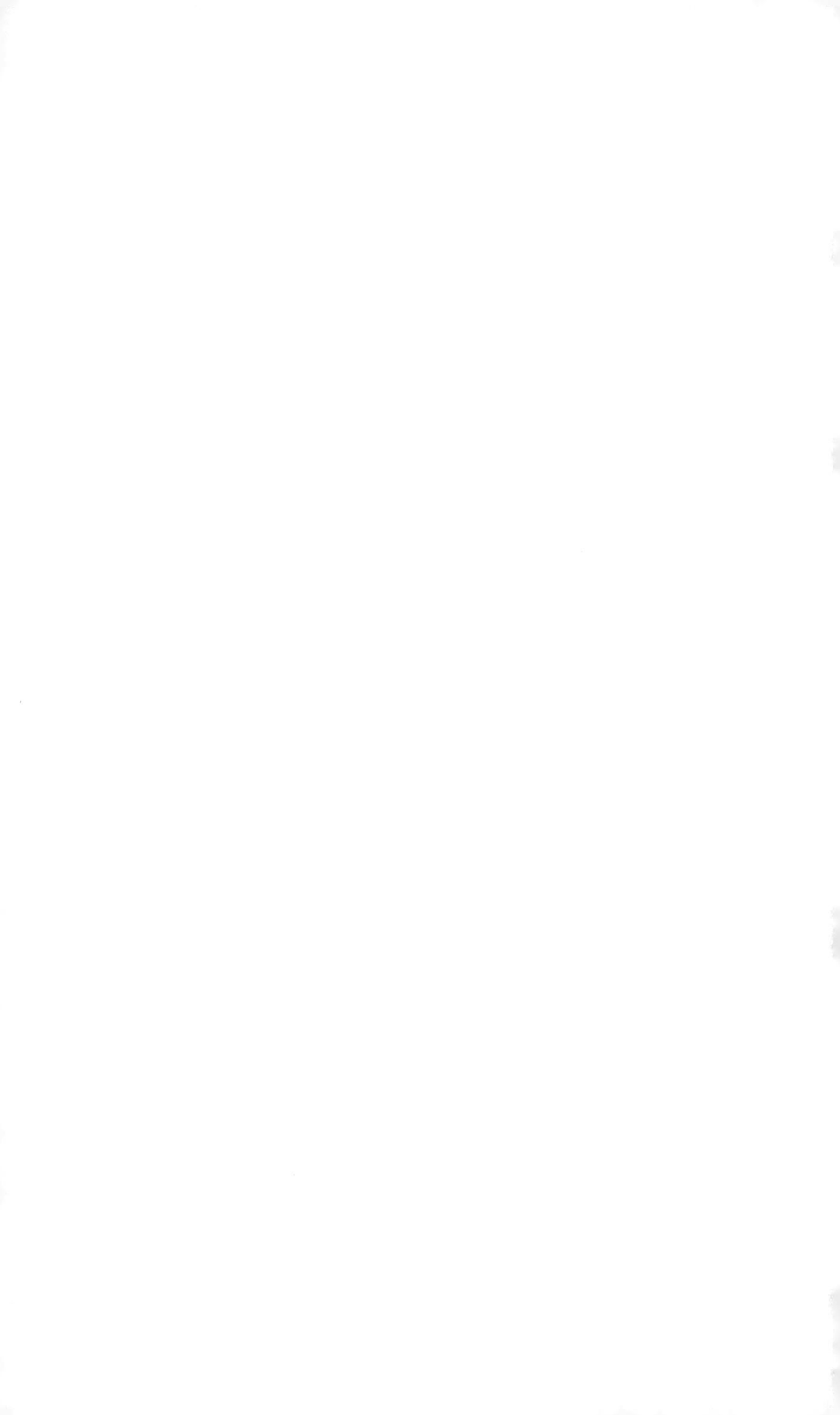

Janna S. Gordon-Elliott
Anna H. Rosen
Editors

Early Career Physician Mental Health and Wellness

A Clinical Casebook

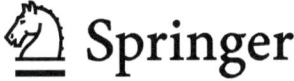 Springer

Editors
Janna S. Gordon-Elliott
Weill Cornell Medical College/
New York-Presbyterian
Hospital
New York, NY
USA

Anna H. Rosen
Weill Cornell Medical College/
New York-Presbyterian
Hospital-Westchester Division
White Plains, NY
USA

ISBN 978-3-030-10951-6   ISBN 978-3-030-10952-3   (eBook)
https://doi.org/10.1007/978-3-030-10952-3

Library of Congress Control Number: 2019933403

This Springer imprint is published by the registered company Springer Nature Switzerland AG
The registered company address is: Gewerbestrasse 11, 6330 Cham, Switzerland

Preface

Young adulthood is a time of substantial transition, growth, risk, and opportunity. Transitioning out of adolescence involves developmental challenges including, but not limited to, establishment of independence, crystallization of personality, navigation of intimate relationships, and laying the groundwork for a career. This stage of life is also the time when psychiatric conditions and other mental health issues often first present, with the possibility of delaying or derailing these developmental milestones. For these reasons, young adulthood is a critical period – one that can set stage for the rest of a lifetime.

Medical trainees (including medical students and residents) and junior attendings are typically young adults. The usual demands of young adulthood can be intensified and aggravated by the specific challenges faced in medical education and the subsequent responsibilities of working as a physician, from work load and work hours to caring for the very sick, to financial debt, and to the pressures of the "culture" of medicine and medical institutions. Generally resilient and competent as a population, physicians in training and early in their careers face substantial stress and often benefit from, or require, psychiatric care. The alternative is grim. Studies estimate that physicians have the highest rate of suicide of any professional group, with almost one suicide daily by a physician [1, 2]. Difficulties may start early, with some estimates indicating that up to one-half of medical students will experience burnout, and more than 10% will have suicidal ideation over a 12-month period [3].

Generally, medical trainees and young physicians have treatable mental health conditions, and early identification and treatment can drastically alter the trajectory of illness and their lives. Despite this, there can be a reluctance to pursue care [5]. The limiting factors abound – time constraints, shame and stigma, and concerns about potential negative impact of a psychiatric illness on one's future career. Psychiatric care during this decisive period can be essential for these individuals, establishing the basis for ongoing mental health and resilience, with implications on future well-being, career success, and professionalism.

Most psychiatrists will at some point be in a position of providing care or consultation to medical trainees and young physicians, even if they do not work specifically for mental health services dedicated to this population, and in so doing will ask to assess and manage complex issues during a dynamic period in their patients' lives. The psychiatric care of these physician-patients must tend to the specific context of healthcare training; the potential hazards of untreated illness on these patients' lives, loved ones, and the profession of medicine; and the characteristic challenges that exist in the treatment of "one of our own." We compiled this casebook to highlight the typical experiences met in the psychiatric treatment of young physicians: from diagnosis to management and from interfacing with the systems that oversee and support these physician-patients to addressing common countertransference responses that arise when a physician treats another physician. Through the use of illustrative cases and relatable discussions, we hope the reader will gain understanding and comfort with treating a variety of mental health issues in physicians and physicians-in-training.

The patients presented in this book were created as fictional cases to reflect the experiences our authors have had with students and junior doctors who have presented to see us – in the therapy office, the emergency room, or the inpatient psychiatric setting. These are patients who may be difficult to treat, but the care of whom can be particularly rewarding. While we explore topics and indications for treatment that are universal – such as burnout, onset of major mental illness, suicide, professionalism issues, and substance use – we hope to emphasize the ways in which managing these conditions in medical students, residents, and junior attendings made these cases uniquely challenging.

Clinical material is drawn from the authors' clinical experience over many years and in different treatment settings, as well as idealized and prototypical diagnostic presentations. All cases presented have been developed by the authors combining characteristics of real individuals as well as fictitious elements. No case presented in this book represents a specific individual; there is no direct association between one of these cases and an individual that our authors have provided care for professionally. First and last names were created and assigned and have no connection to actual patients.

New York, NY, USA   Janna S. Gordon-Elliott
White Plains, NY, USA   Anna H. Rosen

References

1. Frank E, et al. Mortality rates and causes among U.S. physicians. Am J Prev Med. 2000; 19(3):155–9.
2. Center C, Davis M, Detre T, et al. Confronting depression and suicide in physicians: a consensus statement. JAMA. 2003;289(23):3161–6. https://doi.org/10.1001/jama.289.23.3161
3. Dyrbye LN, Thomas MR, Massie FS, et al. Burnout and suicidal ideation among U.S. medical students. Ann Intern Med. 2008;149(5):334–1.
4. Shanafelt TD, Bradley KA, Wipf JE, Back AL. Burnout and self-reported patient care in an internal medicine residency program. Ann Intern Med.2002;136:358–67.
5. Givens JL, Tjia J. Depressed medical students' use of mental health services and barriers to use. Acad Med.2002;77:918–21.

Contents

Contributors

Jonathan Avery, MD Weill Cornell Medical College/New York-Presbyterian Hospital, New York, NY, USA

Shannon G. Caspersen, MD Weill Cornell Medical College, New York, NY, USA

Anna L. Dickerman, MD Weill Cornell Medical College/New York-Presbyterian Hospital, New York, NY, USA

Rebecca Fein, MD Weill Cornell Medical College/New York-Presbyterian Hospital, New York, NY, USA

Elena Friedman, MD Weill Cornell Medical College/New York-Presbyterian Hospital, New York, NY, USA

Liliya Gershengoren, MD, MPH Weill Cornell Medical College/New York-Presbyterian Hospital, New York, NY, USA

Janna S. Gordon-Elliott, MD Weill Cornell Medical College/New York-Presbyterian Hospital, New York, NY, USA

Alyson Gorun, MD Weill Cornell Medical College/New York-Presbyterian Hospital, New York, NY, USA

Christopher R. Green, MD Weill Cornell Medical College/New York-Presbyterian Hospital, New York, NY, USA

Bernadine H. Han, MD, MS New York University School of Medicine/Bellevue Hospital Center, New York, NY, USA

David Hankins, MD, MEd Weill Cornell Medical College/New York-Presbyterian Hospital, New York, NY, USA

Kristopher A. Kast, MD Weill Cornell Medical College/New York-Presbyterian Hospital, New York, NY, USA

Daniel Knoepflmacher, MD, MFA Weill Cornell Medical College/New York-Presbyterian Hospital, New York, NY, USA

Nisha Mehta-Naik, MD Weill Cornell Medical College/New York-Presbyterian Hospital, New York, NY, USA

Anna Miari, MD Weill Cornell Medical College/New York-Presbyterian Hospital, New York, NY, USA

Julie Penzner, MD Weill Cornell Medical College/New York-Presbyterian Hospital, New York, NY, USA

Anna H. Rosen, MD Weill Cornell Medical College/New York-Presbyterian Hospital-Westchester Division, White Plains, NY, USA

Renee Saenger, MD Weill Cornell Medical College/New York-Presbyterian Hospital-Westchester Division, White Plains, NY, USA

Anna Salajegheh, MD Weill Cornell Medical College/New York-Presbyterian Hospital, New York, NY, USA

Charles W. Shaffer, MD Weill Cornell Medical College/New York-Presbyterian Hospital, New York, NY, USA

Jess Zonana, MD Weill Cornell Medical College/New York-Presbyterian Hospital, New York, NY, USA

Gwen L. Zornberg, MD, MSc, ScD Weill Cornell Medical College/New York-Presbyterian Hospital, New York, NY, USA

Chapter 1
The Case of Joseph Martinez: A Medical Student with Mania

Shannon G. Caspersen

Case

Joseph Martinez, a 26-year-old, third-year medical student at a medical school in a small city, hoping to match in neurosurgery, presented to the psychiatric emergency department (ED) of the affiliated hospital with security officers from the medical school.

Joseph, who had never been treated for any psychiatric condition in the past, had been escorted from the medical school library to the ED when he refused to leave the library at closing time (11 p.m.). The security officers explained that they had found him pacing up and down the stacks mumbling medical-sounding words under his breath and insisting to them that he had to stay until he had "solved the equation." The officers told Joseph that if he would not leave, they would call the police, at which time he became loud and physically threatening, shouting that he had been commissioned by the surgeon general to find a cure for kidney failure by solving an obscure equation that had been lost to medical

S. G. Caspersen, MD (✉)
Weill Cornell Medical College, New York, NY, USA
e-mail: contact@shannoncasepersenmd.com

© Springer Nature Switzerland AG 2019
J. S. Gordon-Elliott, A. H. Rosen (eds.), *Early Career Physician Mental Health and Wellness*,
https://doi.org/10.1007/978-3-030-10952-3_1

history until he himself unearthed it during his internal medicine rotation, the shelf exam for which was the following morning.

The security officers, both of whom had worked many shifts in the affiliated hospital's psychiatric ED, recognized in Joseph the pressured speech and grandiosity that they had seen in some patients in the psychiatric ED in the past, so called for backup and escorted him there rather than calling the police.

On presentation to the ED, Joseph appeared disheveled (several days' beard growth, dark circles under his eyes, oily hair, and food stains on his shirt and white coat). When approached by the second-year psychiatry resident working in the ED, Joseph recognized him and said, "I know you from med school. You were a fourth year when I was a first year. It's always the dumbest med students who match in psychiatry. You would never understand the level of medical complexity I am engaged in right now. Get me the attending."

The resident, maintaining a neutral tone, explained that the attending would be there in the morning but that for now Joseph could perhaps describe how he had come to be in the ED.

Joseph's speech was indeed pressured as he described how he had been awake for the last 3 nights attempting to solve "the equation to end ESRD [end stage-kidney disease] and dialysis forever." He stated proudly that, prior to those 3 nights, he had done three overnight shifts in a row on the medicine wards by taking shifts for two of his classmates, in hopes of getting extra credit on his internal medicine rotation. He stated that he was confident that he would "ace the shelf exam" the following morning, provided that he was released immediately from the ED to finish studying for it. He was so confident, he said, that he felt he could devote several hours to solving the equation, as requested by the surgeon general, before sitting down to study for the shelf.

When interviewed by the attending psychiatrist in the ED, he presented similarly, with pressured speech, increased energy and goal-directed activity, and grandiosity.

Collateral obtained from Joseph's internal medicine course director confirmed that Joseph's behavior had changed over the last week, and the director was planning to contact the medical school dean the following morning, after the shelf exam, to express concern.

Joseph denied ever having had any psychiatric problems in the past or in the present. He stated that if he were not released from the ED immediately, he would "punch out" the attending and the resident and also sue the hospital.

The attending determined that the second-year resident, who had indeed known Joseph socially in medical school, should not manage the case in the ED. Joseph refused to answer any questions that did not directly pertain to his being discharged from the ED, refused medication offered, and refused admission to the inpatient psychiatric unit at the hospital, stating, "my psych rotation isn't until the end of the year—I'm saving the easy ones for the end."

Joseph was determined to be a risk to others, given his threatening statements and physical aggression, and a risk to himself given his having not slept in at least 6 nights and his highly irritable state. He was hospitalized involuntarily.

The ED attending was also the inpatient unit attending, but Joseph was assigned to a different resident, who he had not known previously. He was able to view this resident as his physician, rather than as a peer, which helped him assume the patient role more easily on the unit than he had been able to in the ED. He remained dismissive of the attending and refused to discuss anything other than his discharge during rounds but would speak with the inpatient resident individually. They would walk down the ward hallways while talking, so that Joseph could pace, as he had been doing since his arrival, and the resident could take history. The resident was able to glean that Joseph had had episodes of depression in high school and college, but had never sought treatment, and the episodes had self-resolved. He learned that Joseph's mother had major depressive disorder and that his paternal grandfather had been institutionalized following a "nervous breakdown" for many years. The resident was able to convince Joseph to produce a urine sample, which was negative for substances of abuse, and Joseph reported that he never used drugs, licit or illicit, and had never had more than three drinks at a time, about once per month.

Joseph denied ever having had suicidal ideation, engaging in self-injuring behavior, or committing violence toward others.

Principles of Diagnosis and Management

Diagnosis

The most appropriate diagnosis for Joseph is bipolar I disorder, severe, current episode manic, with psychotic features [1]. He is exhibiting a discrete period (approximately 1 week based on his report of 6 sleepless nights and a change in behavior noted by the course director over the last week) of elevated and irritable mood, grandiosity (believing he has been commissioned by the surgeon general to solve one of medicine's more significant ailments), decreased need for sleep, pressured speech, and increased goal-directed activity (extra shifts, all-night studying). His physical aggression and erratic behavior are interfering with his functioning. His history of depression, though untreated, supports a diagnosis of bipolar disorder, as does his family history of mood disorders, including his grandfather's "nervous breakdown" which may have represented a manic or depressive episode. The fact that his manic episode was severe enough to necessitate a hospitalization qualifies Joseph for a diagnosis of bipolar I.

As this was an initial psychiatric presentation, the inpatient treatment team considered a wide differential diagnosis, including substance-induced bipolar or psychotic disorders, primary psychotic disorders, and personality disorders. The negative urine test and the lack of substance use history aside from monthly moderate drinking make a substance-induced manic episode less likely (though the urine sample was not produced immediately, and therefore would not reveal the use of substances that do not appear in urine outside of a very short time window, or those substances that may not be detected by the particular toxicology assay). The prominence of mood symptoms in addition to the psychotic symptoms prioritizes a bipolar disorder over a pure psychotic disorder. The substantial change in mood and behavior over a short (1-week) period makes a personality disorder less likely. Further collateral obtained from Joseph's dean and from his parents clarified that he had not exhibited prodromal symptoms consistent with an emerging psychotic disorder, was not known to use any substances (including psychoactive prescriptions that could induce mania, such as stimulants or corticosteroids), and was not known to have previously displayed any of the behaviors that were present in the week leading up to his hospitalization. His parents did note that he had been a "moody" teenager who could spend several days in bed without showering. These behaviors, which his parents at the time attributed to "typical teenagehood," could have represented untreated major depression.

Management

The most important initial treatment for bipolar mania is mood-stabilizing medication. Ideally, Joseph would have received medication from the ED, but since he was refusing and did not pose *immediate* bodily harm to himself or others in the ED, he was not given intramuscular medication. On the inpatient unit, where he quickly developed a rapport with the resident, he was offered oral valproate, which was titrated to a therapeutic blood level, with quetiapine at bedtime to restore a normal sleep pattern, which in turn diminished the mania. Lithium would have been an option for mood stabilization as well, but given Joseph's psychotic preoccupation with ESRD, he refused a medication that was potentially nephrotoxic.

Once a patient with mania begins to stabilize, the patient may be more receptive to group and individual therapy, with a focus on safety, discharge planning, and recurrence prevention.

Principles for Doctors Treating Doctors

Some of the symptoms and behaviors that can lead to, exacerbate, or represent mania are glorified in medical student culture. Being high-energy, being able to stay up all night to study or do shifts, and engaging in highly focused goal-directed behavior are not only desirable in medical students—they are requisite. In an individual like Joseph, who is genetically predisposed to bipolar disorder and is in the age range at which a first episode characteristically occurs, the demands and pressures of medical school can make the symptoms he was experiencing seem, at least at first, to be normative. His taking on extra shifts and staying late in the library could be experienced by him and by his peers and instructors as typical of an ambitious and high-achieving medical student, or, in med school slang, a "gunner." Even his delusions of grandeur—that he has unearthed an obscure equation and must solve it at the behest of the surgeon general in order to cure ESRD—are ego-syntonic with the medical student's idealized calling to achieve, innovate, and save lives. Perhaps Joseph would have had more insight into his mood disturbance at an earlier stage if it had not been aligned so closely with the goals and values of a budding medical professional.

Once Joseph was brought to the ED by concerned security staff, his identity changed from grandiose hero-physician, saving the world from ESRD, to patient. He found himself in the far from grandiose position of being a patient on a medical service of a specialty he seemed to disrespect and under the care of a physician whom he regarded as a peer—and an inferior one at that. We do not know what his attitude toward psychiatry and this particular resident/former schoolmate was prior to his manic episode, but there was likely a degree of disdain pre-mania that was exaggerated or revealed in the context of the illness.

As Joseph's valproate level became therapeutic, he was able to discuss how he experienced his hospitalization as a fall from grace — from a "AOA-track neurosurg-matcher" to a "nutcase on the psych ward." On the one hand, he expressed fear that his "brain was broken" and he would need to drop out of medical school, and on the other, he demanded that his psych rotation be changed to an away-rotation at a hospital in another city, because he was ashamed of being a patient and of how he had behaved toward the ED resident and the attending when he was manic.

While gently addressing these all-or-nothing, black-and-white statements with techniques of cognitive behavioral therapy, the inpatient clinicians considered, among themselves, the quite realistic risks of Joseph's continuing on an ambitious medical career. For example, there were good reasons to be thoughtful about future lifestyle demands, such as lack of sleep and changes in sleep schedule, which are risk factors for mania in patients with bipolar disorder. If he were to choose to match in neurosurgery, Joseph's shift schedule as a medical student, resident, and attending might increase his chances of manic relapses. Side effects of some mood stabilizers, such as tremor, could also be problematic for a career as a surgeon. Lastly, though Joseph denied any problematic substance use, his academic and clinical ambitions and the possibility for cognitive dulling that could occur with valproate or another mood stabilizer put him at risk for stimulant use or misuse, which could in turn exacerbate another episode of mania. The team chose to delay exploration of these longer-term issues, deciding that these concerns might be better addressed on an outpatient basis, once Joseph had established rapport with an outpatient psychiatrist, with whom he could strategize about the ways to keep himself stable and optimize his mental health over time.

Joseph's different transference experiences toward specific psychiatrists and his transference toward psychiatry in general would likely elicit negative countertransference responses in his treating psychiatrists, both negative (his former schoolmate who he devalued in the ED) and positive (his inpatient resident, whom he idealized and who might feel like Joseph's savior and the "only one" who can connect with him). For the resident evaluating and working with Joseph, the similarities between them could lead to overidentification, potentially subtly affecting the resident's behavior—perhaps by minimizing Joseph's symptoms or by responding to Joseph in a judgmental or punitive way. Both of which responses may be related to unconscious anxiety generated by imagining that something like this could happen to the resident. Careful and attentive supervision from the attending for the resident treating this patient is not only essential but may also allow for a tremendous educational experience and significant professional growth for the resident. This case also highlights how the relationship between non-psychiatrist physicians and their psychiatrists is undoubtedly affected by attitudes and beliefs that physicians hold about their own specialties and those of others; the non-psychiatrist patient will experience the treatment with a psychiatrist in part through the lens of his attitudes (both positive and negative) about psychiatry, and the psychiatrist's ideas about the specialty of the non-psychiatrist patient will be part of the psychiatrist's experience. The psychiatrist must be attentive to this process and—as indicated—address beliefs and biases actively, either individually (e.g., in supervision, therapy, or self-exploration) or directly in the dynamic with the patient. Physicians in other fields may think about personal psychiatric illness in a very different way, sometimes specific to their chosen specialty, than the psychiatrist treating them does. For Joseph, his goal to treat the brain as a surgeon, in a mechanical way, is a particularly interesting juxtaposition to the perspective of the psychiatrist, who for the most part treats the brain in a decidedly less mechanical way. In the treatment, the psychiatrist can work with some of these perspectives as not an obstacle but a way of engaging the physician patient.

Outcome

Joseph returned to school after a medical leave for his hospitalization, followed by a week at home with his parents during which he studied for his shelf exam in internal medicine. He took the exam upon his return to school and obtained an average score. He worked with his new outpatient psychiatrist to process what it meant to him to achieve an average, rather than superlative score, as he was used to doing. With the assistance of student mental health leadership and the dean's office, Joseph's rotation schedule was rearranged so that he could do electives and non-call rotations earlier, saving more intensive rotations for later in the year. He remained stable on valproate, with occasional use of quetiapine when he had trouble sleeping or needed to go to sleep in the morning after an overnight shift. He discussed his desire to continue to pursue a residency in neurosurgery with his psychiatrist and ultimately determined that he would take a year off from medical school to do a research fellowship before deciding on a specialty. His psychiatrist emphasized the importance of medication adherence and checked blood levels of valproate more frequently than the recommended every 4–6 months, given the high stakes of the patient falling below a therapeutic blood level. He remained mostly side-effect-free through his first year of valproate treatment.

Pearls
- Lifestyles conducive to manic-like behavior can mask and/or exacerbate mania
- Hierarchical relationships between medical trainees and professionals, as well as between members of different specialties, can arouse unique transference-countertransference reactions
- Effect and side effect profiles of mood stabilizers need to be taken into account when choosing medications for particular patients with bipolar disorders, according to their lifestyles and life goals.

Reference

1. American Psychiatric Association. Diagnostic and statistical manual of mental disorders. 5th ed. Arlington: American Psychiatric Publishing; 2013.

Suggested Reading

Avery JD, Barnhill JW, editors. Co-occurring mental illness and substance use disorders. Arlington: American Psychiatric Publishing, Chapter 3: Depressive and bipolar disorders; 2018. p. 25–38.
Viktorin A, Ryden E, Thase ME, et al. The risk of treatment-emergent mania with methylphenidate in bipolar disorder. Am J Psychiatry. 2017;174:341–8.

Chapter 2
The Case of Monica Khuma: More than Borderline Difficulties

Anna H. Rosen

Case

Monica, a 24-year-old second year medical student at a mid-Atlantic urban medical school, presented to Dr. Noyes, a psychiatrist in practice for 15 years, with the chief complaint: "I was told to come here." Dr. Noyes was the fourth psychiatrist that Monica had seen since the beginning of high school and felt that each one "failed her." Nonetheless, Monica's mother urged her to seek treatment after making a suicidal statement to her over the phone. Monica arrived on time for her appointment with Dr. Noyes – put together and poised she glided into the office – deliberately avoiding the gaze of the other patients in the waiting area. She began speaking without prompting from Dr. Noyes. She shared her difficulties with a rehearsed quality, punctuated with professional jargon. She endorsed a lifelong preoccupation with perfectionism, difficulty making and keeping friends, and a sense of shame related to her father's alcoholism. Monica's difficulty cultivating close friendships fueled an intensity about academic achievement. Medical school was the culmination of

A. H. Rosen, MD (✉)
Weill Cornell Medical College/New York-Presbyterian Hospital-Westchester Division, White Plains, NY, USA
e-mail: ash9006@med.cornell.edu

© Springer Nature Switzerland AG 2019   11
J. S. Gordon-Elliott, A. H. Rosen (eds.), *Early Career Physician Mental Health and Wellness*,
https://doi.org/10.1007/978-3-030-10952-3_2

years of focus and hard work. While part of her was wary of pursuing medicine, she knew that she liked school, thrived within structured environments, and imagined she would be among driven, like-minded individuals. Monica matriculated into medical school right after college.

Since high school, Monica was evaluated by three psychiatrists but consistently felt misunderstood adding that she was "far more intelligent than any of these doctors." Dr. Noyes interjected – "You are right, you may have been more intelligent than them." This unnerved and confused Monica and she struggled to pivot from Dr. Noyes's interjection. Part of Monica's difficulty related to her rigidity. With the start of medical school, among classmates who were of varying ages and life experiences, Monica struggled to balance her competitiveness with her wish to connect to peers. She described an intensification of her baseline irritability and feelings of emptiness. As a way to release her anger, she scratch and then cut herself, first on her forearms and then over her inner thighs. At first, this was a rare occurrence, but over time, Monica's self-injury escalated to almost every day.

During the first four weeks of medical school, Monica thought about suicide for the first time. She was studying for an anatomy quiz in a lounge on the eighth floor. She looked out of the eighth floor window, considered how she could go about opening it, and imagined the fall. Monica did not open the window, but over the year since then, in more desperate moments, she would sit beside this window as though she was studying and imagined her death. She said that she did not think about the impact that her suicide would have on her family. A week before meeting Dr. Noyes, while on the phone with her mother, Monica revealed intermittent suicidal thoughts with the plan to jump out of the eighth floor study room window.

Monica denied feeling like she had a drinking problem but did acknowledge that that once every one to two months, she would drink six or more drinks in a night. Typically, she would start while out with friends, but not uncommonly drink more on her own later. She explained that this could be triggered by negative feelings, such as feeling lonely or overwhelmed or rejected by a perceived social or romantic slight.

In the initial evaluation session, Dr. Noyes assessed Monica for current suicidality, and Monica denied having any thought of suicide. Dr. Noyes reviewed Monica's upcoming responsibilities – wondering about her potential vulnerability around sick patients. Monica did not have any clinical encounters scheduled. They set up a time to meet later in the week.

Principles of Diagnosis and Management

Diagnosis

The most appropriate diagnosis for Monica is borderline personality disorder (BPD). Patients with BPD suffer from unstable self-image and concurrent difficulty managing their affect and behaviors. The DSM-5 diagnostic criteria for BPD include "a pervasive pattern of instability of interpersonal relationships, self-image, and affects, and marked impulsivity, beginning by early adulthood and present in a variety of contexts [1]." With further evaluation of Monica's difficulties, Dr. Noyes appreciated a pattern of unstable and intense interpersonal relationships, a lack of self-awareness (specifically, an inability to see herself as others see her), a chronic experience of emptiness, impulsive self-destructive behaviors, and recurrent suicidal thoughts and actions.

While Monica clearly exhibited symptoms of BPD, Dr. Noyes's differential included major depressive disorder, anxiety disorder (panic disorder and generalized anxiety disorder), bipolar disorder, alcohol use disorder, and cannabis use disorder. Critical to Dr. Noyes's understanding was the chronicity of some of her symptoms (i.e., identity diffusion, lack of stable self-image) punctuated by periods of mood lability, impulsivity, and suicidal ideation. In contrast to a major depressive episode, Monica's symptoms did not present with significant neurovegetative symptoms. She was able to maintain her activities of daily living and did not think of herself as sad. In contrast, she described feeling "nothing" or anger. She denied panic or irrational fears suggestive of an anxiety disorder but reported feeling chronically "on edge." Unlike a patient in the midst of a hypomanic or manic state, she was not elevated nor did she present with accompanying grandiosity, limitless energy, or sleep disturbance. Monica reported drinking alcoholic beverages once a month but when she did would frequently drink 3–4 drinks alone and sometimes would blackout at the end of the night. She did not see this as problematic or potentially dangerous. For some with borderline personality disorder, alcohol or other substance use can magnify insecurities, impulsivity, and mood lability.

Management and Treatment

The mainstay of treatment for BPD is the combination psychotherapy and pharmacotherapy. Therapies including dialectical behavioral therapy (DBT), transference focused psychotherapy (TFP), and mentalization-based treatment (MBT) have been developed specifically to treat patients suffering from BPD. At their core, each of these psychotherapies works with treatment contracts, strategies to address premature termination, crisis interventions, and a focus on interpersonal awareness and therapeutic alliance.

While Monica did not fulfill criteria for a comorbid mood, anxiety, or substance use disorder, the medications frequently used to address these issues – antidepressants, anxiolytics, and mood stabilizers – can be beneficial to patients with BPD. The greatest benefit of pharmacological options is when there is a specific symptom to target with medication such as mood lability. Monica, for example, benefited from escitalopram – a selective serotonin reuptake inhibitor (SSRI) which helped brighten her mood and relieve some of her anxiety and restlessness.

Principles for Doctors Treating Doctors

Upon initial presentation, Monica expressed ambivalence about her difficulties, demonstrating a profound lack of self-awareness and perpetuating her anger that others psychiatrists failed to help her address her difficulties. She experienced the latter as humiliating, and in her mind, it delayed her ability to access treatment. During Dr. Noyes's initial sessions with Monica, she clarified Monica's symptoms. She thought about the ways it was going to be difficult for Monica to be a patient and the ways Monica would struggle treating patients and managing their needs as a medical student and later a physician. Central to alliance formation was a neutral and empathic stance which Dr. Noyes hoped would model boundaries and caretaking for Monica.

Dr. Noyes summarized her findings after three sessions. She diagnosed Monica with BPD and recommended twice weekly psychotherapy. Monica was upset by her diagnosis. Borderline was a word she heard thrown around the hospital for unsavory and difficult patients. Dr. Noyes asked her to tell her more about this. Monica shared an experience from her first year in medical school while she was shadowing a medicine resident on an inpatient service. The patient in the resident's care threw a tray of food at a nurse. The resident's pager starting buzzing while he was in the midst of coaxing a patient who wanted to leave against medical advice to stay in the hospital. Monica followed the resident into the hallway and watched him throw his hands up in exasperation as he rhetorically asked if "these people could just get locked up on psych." He then gave Monica his pager and asked her to "deal with it." Monica recalled to Dr. Noyes how she felt at a loss. She remembered feeling unskilled and furious. She started scratching her forearm until she noticed the resident staring at her arm with some concern. Monica could not decide where to direct her ire. She was angry with the patient, imagining her as ungrateful and disruptive and now causing more work for Monica. Simultaneously, she was enraged by the resident's response, wondering how he could behave so dismissively toward his patients.

She imagined herself as a resident in a few years. She identified with both the dysregulated patient and the disparaging resident. Unable to separate her experience from the "bad" patient, she internalized the experience as a reflection of her own emotional dysregulation, reinforcing her experience of herself as a poorly behaved, angry person. That night, confused by the day's events and uncomfortable with her emotions, Monica continued scratching and then cut herself. She was relieved that her scars would be covered with long sleeves and her white coat. Recalling this in Dr. Noyes's office, she felt shamed and "outed" with Dr. Noyes's diagnosis Dr. Noyes validated Monica's experience as well as the toll placed on her to "deal" with a patient who was clearly struggling and unable to articulate her needs effectively. She asked Monica to imagined herself as the physician in this episode and how she would have managed the patient's care and her own affect. The patient was given medication by the time Monica arrived at her bedside and was practically asleep. She revealed that she was relieved that she did not have to "deal" with the situation and angry that the patient's needs seemed ignored. Dr. Noyes wondered about Monica's inability to control the events and subsequent attack on herself. She asked if the team met with the patient after the incident. Monica wasn't sure. Cautiously, Dr. Noyes offered an interpretation of the scenario: Monica identified with the treatment team's frustration as well as the patient's aggression. She felt as though she had to pick "sides" and was unable to consolidate her experience, feeling so overwhelmed with her own and other's affect that her only recourse was to attack herself.

Monica and Dr. Noyes were scheduled to meet twice weekly with treatment organized around a mutually agreed upon contract adhering to the model of transference focused psychotherapy. From the onset of treatment, Monica struggled with attendance. When Monica canceled appointments at the last minute (as was frequently the case), the next session was focused on her absence. Several months into treatment, after a string of repeated absences, Monica presented as particularly irritable. Anticipating Dr. Noyes's focus on her most recent canceled appointment, she began: "Can we speak about something else? When I am not here it's because I am taking care of patients" adding "and my cutting is getting much worse." Dr. Noyes validated Monica's hard work but needed to reflect transferentially on Monica's anger. In the session it was directed at Dr. Noyes. Outside of session she directed it on herself. Dr. Noyes wondered how this impacted Monica's interactions in the hospital and ability to deliver patient care. Dr. Noyes pointed out that her difficulty setting up boundaries was impacting her own care – both with repeated cancelations and intensification of self-harm. Dr. Noyes recalled Monica's experience earlier in the year with the dysregulated "borderline" patient. Overidentifying with the rageful patient and unsympathetic resident prompted her own attack on herself. Monica took a deep breath. Reflecting, "if I could have taken a deep breath in that moment, I would have been more useful, or at the very least wouldn't have started scratching my arms in front of my resident." This was a subtle but an important boundary that Monica could access in the future.

Monica's challenges were multi-tiered. She presented with an illness that can be difficult to identify, difficult to treat, and frequently misunderstood. Even among colleagues in the medical community, borderline is used as an adjective or, worst yet, an expletive connoting challenging, unsatisfied, and time-consuming patients. When borderline is used as a pejorative descriptor, this highlights providers' sense of futility managing medically challenging and affectively dysregulated patients. At the same time, this minimizes the psychological experiences of their patients and a disavowal of treatment for others with mood lability, interpersonal difficulties, and those diagnosed with borderline personality disorder. In treatment, psychoeducation around the word, usage, and diagnostic criteria of borderline personality disorder delineates the experience of providing care for medically and psychiatrically ill patients – a challenge all future physicians will encounter – and seeing oneself as having a treatable illness. To this end, Monica's identification with this patient's rage and impulsivity stood as a barrier for engagement in treatment, rather than a motivation to understand and contain her own difficulties. Monica internalized the resident's resentment toward borderline patients and imagined her own difficulties met with similar capitulation from providers. Psychoeducation around these issues as well as orienting a patient to a structured treatment with goals and expectations is therapeutic and instructive.

Dr. Noyes employed the same strategy in her organization of Monica's treatment. Their treatment contract addressed safety (self-injury and suicidal ideation), treatment-interfering activities (attendance, alcohol use), and Monica's interpersonal challenges. Each session opened with the focus on Monica's treatment contract. This can be challenging for patients with borderline personality disorder with particular vulnerabilities to shame and perceived criticism. The focus on the contract, however, facilitates discussion of Monica's most central difficulties in a contained environment. Other modalities such as DBT incorporate diary cards and treatment hierarchies to orient the patient and provider to the most pressing issues for their sessions. These strategies address resistance in treatment and acknowledge the difficulty patients with borderline personality disorder have managing their internal emotional organization. Organization and consistency in treatment offer a sense of control for the borderline patient when exploring the most affectively charged subjects. The result is both therapeutic and supportive. Monica's progress relied upon her acceptance of the role of a patient and subsequently to see herself as someone worthy of care and attention from a physician – the same kind of care she imagined giving to future patients.

Outcome

Monica continued to see Dr. Noyes twice weekly for the duration of medical school. She struggled with a sense of shame relating to "needing" treatment and was able to express relief that Dr. Noyes prescribed the treatment. With an emphasis on identification of emotional states, consolidating disparate feelings and behaviors and creating boundaries for self-care, Monica matured as an individual and caretaker. Two years into treatment while deciding upon her specialty, Monica proposed pursuing psychiatry. Dr. Noyes's initial response was pride, feeling as though she succeeded as a clinician. Aware of her own countertransference and wish to help as well as Monica's tendency to overidentify with those in her midst, Dr. Noyes addressed this in the treatment. Monica expressed empathy for psychiatric patients. She related to their vulnerabilities and felt as though she could "advocate" for them. Dr. Noyes asked Monica if this was something she thought she would enjoy or a way of protecting herself. Monica was able to reflect and consider the skills that she wanted to use daily; advocating for psychiatric patients was not isolated to the work of psychiatrists. She thought about what she wanted and what interested and challenged her. Ultimately, she applied and matched in internal medicine. Her experience was less colored by shame and she felt hopeful about her future.

Pearls
- It is important to establish a contract to frame and organize the treatment with expectations around: meeting times, frequency of sessions, events that occur between sessions, steps to take in the event of an emergency, and clear expectations around potential notification of administration. This clarity of structure will contrast with patient's internal chaos.
- Neutrality as a treater. Patients with borderline personality disorder typically present to treatment with accumulated negative, invalidating experiences, and to protect against this experience, their impulse is to devalue and/or idealize the treater. A neutral, empathic provider can most aptly guide a patient with borderline personality disorder to develop a cohesive self-representation.
- Clarification of goals and expectations of treatment. The more psychoeducation the better – this offers clarity and containment of affective states – elements that patients with borderline personality disorder are likely to lack in their internal lives.
- Screen for co-occurring psychiatric and substance use disorders.

Reference

1. American Psychiatric Association. Diagnostic and statistical manual of mental disorders. 5th ed. Arlington: American Psychiatric Publishing; 2013.

Suggested Reading

Bateman A, Fonagy P. Treatment of borderline personality disorder with psychoanalytically oriented partial hospitalization: an 18-month follow-up. Am J Psychiatr. 2001;158:36–42.

Clarkin JF, Yeomans FE, Kernberg OF. Psychotherapy for borderline personality. New York: Wiley; 1999.

De Groot ER, Verheul R, Trijsburg RW. An integrative perspective on psychotherapeutic treatments for borderline personality disorders. J Personal Disord. 2008;22:332–52.

Linehan MM. Cognitive behavioral treatment of borderline personality disorder. New York: Guilford; 1993.

Linehan MM. The skills training manual for treating borderline personality disorder. New York: Guilford; 1993.

Ripoll LH. Clinical psychopharmacology of borderline personality disorder: an update on the available evidence in light of the diagnostic and statistical manual of mental disorders - 5. Curr Opin Psychiatry. 2012;25:52–8.

Chapter 3
The Case of James Dire: The Problem with Panic

Liliya Gershengoren

Case

James Dire, a 26-year-old third year medical student at a northeast urban medical school, presented to Dr. Waser, a psychiatrist with over 20 years of experience working in the medical school mental health clinic, with the chief complaint: "No offense, but I really don't think that this is psychiatric." James went on to explain that he had already seen multiple medical providers after at least three visits to the medical emergency room and was finally encouraged to seek out psychiatric assessment and treatment. He felt that this referral was made in error and that his symptoms were not being taken seriously by his other physicians. James spoke in a confident and determined manner as he painstakingly described multiple misgivings about having been asked to speak with a psychiatrist; in contrast, he was notably vague in his recounting of the symptoms which had prompted his initial visits to the emergency room and consultations with multiple primary care providers and specialists.

L. Gershengoren, MD, MPH (✉)
Weill Cornell Medical College/New York-Presbyterian Hospital, New York, NY, USA
e-mail: lig9056@med.cornell.edu

© Springer Nature Switzerland AG 2019   21
J. S. Gordon-Elliott, A. H. Rosen (eds.), *Early Career Physician Mental Health and Wellness*,
https://doi.org/10.1007/978-3-030-10952-3_3

Dr. Waser gently encouraged James to describe his symptoms, and after several subtle prompts, James explained that he had repeatedly experienced what he believed to be symptoms of a "heart attack," adding vehemently "that none of the doctors could accurately diagnose." His symptoms began during his first clerkship, internal medicine, during the morning rounds with the medical team. He experienced a sudden onset of dizziness and heart palpitations. He also felt very weak with significant vague abdominal discomfort and shaking in his upper extremities. His resident noticed that James appeared pale and diaphoretic and told him to go sit down and rest. James recalled feeling scared that he was dying and completely losing control of the situation. His father had passed away from a heart attack only 2 years prior, and James was certain that he was experiencing cardiac symptoms. James decided to go to the emergency room immediately. After a thorough physical examination, the emergency room physician said that it was likely anxiety and discharged James with follow-up with his primary care physician.

To James' dismay, his attacks had waxed and waned over the next 6 months and, while always unpredictable, had typically recurred during work hours in front of his medical colleagues. At times, his episodes were characterized by chest discomfort as well as the sensation of a racing or pounding heart. He also experienced shortness of breath, feelings of detachment, and numbness in his extremities. James began to feel anxious about the possibility of another attack especially in a situation that would be both professionally embarrassing and where it would be challenging to obtain emergent medical help. These episodes were unpredictable, which was very unsettling to James, who always prided himself on his ability to remain calm and collected in the face of uncertainty. James was certain that there was a medical explanation for his symptoms and sought out appointments with his primary care physician and subsequently demanded referrals to a cardiologist and a neurologist. The specialists who evaluated James performed more tests, but they all ultimately concluded, to James' consternation, that his symptoms were better described as panic or "anxiety attacks." James finally accepted a referral to Dr. Waser but only to "prove that I'm not insane."

As part of the initial evaluation, Dr. Waser assessed for the presence of mood symptoms and any changes in sleep and appetite, all of which James denied. They reviewed James' medical history, which was unremarkable. James also denied taking any herbal or over-the-counter supplements. He denied significant alcohol use or any illicit drug use. He laughed when he explained that at this point he was even avoiding drinking any caffeinated beverages as they could trigger a sensation of heart palpitations which was too reminiscent of his panic attacks.

At this point in his medical school curriculum, James had elective and vacation time scheduled which left him with a relatively flexible schedule. They agreed to meet once again the following week to discuss diagnosis and treatment plan in greater detail.

Principles of Diagnosis and Management

Diagnosis

The most appropriate diagnosis for James is panic disorder. Panic disorder typically develops in young adulthood but can also develop in other age groups and may be underdiagnosed in the adolescent and geriatric populations. Patients with panic disorder endorse acute episodes of anxiety associated with perceptions of impending doom. Episodes can vary from several events occurring during the day or scattered throughout the year. While an episode of intense anxiety can last from minutes to hours, discreet panic attacks rarely last more than an hour and typically reach a crescendo of symptoms within 10 minutes. Panic disorder is diagnosed when an individual has experienced recurrent panic attacks, and there is at least a 1-month period following a panic attack that is characterized by either persistent concern or worry about having another panic attack or changes in behavior to avoid having a panic attack. Panic disorder should be distinguished from panic attacks occurring as a result of a medication or other substances or a medical disorder [1]. A careful substance use history is essential in a diagnostic evaluation.

Panic disorder commonly co-occurs with other psychiatric conditions such as agoraphobia, social phobia, and specific phobia. About two-third of patients diagnosed with panic disorder experience episodes of panic attacks concurrently with or after the onset of major depression. Patients describe unexpected or unexplained panic attacks, while others experience panic attacks with recognizable patterns or due to known stimuli. Dr. Waser recognized that James' pattern of avoiding caffeinated beverages due to concerns that they would trigger symptoms similar to his panic attacks, as well as his reported anxiety over having future panic attacks, was an important diagnostic theme.

Based on the history gathered, and a review of the extensive medical testing James had received, Dr. Waser felt quite confident in a diagnosis of panic disorder. His differential diagnosis for James included generalized anxiety disorder (GAD), specific and social phobias, and illness anxiety disorder. Differentiation from other anxiety disorders can be challenging. It was important for Dr. Waser to identify that James' reported anxiety was specific to having another panic attack and not attached to other situations or events (i.e., specific or social phobias). Patients with GAD similarly experience physical symptoms associated with anxiety, but they typically describe anxiety and physical symptoms that emerge and dissipate very slowly as compared to panic attacks (though patients with GAD may also have panic attacks, and can be diagnosed, if all criteria are met, with co-occurring panic disorder), and they commonly report a more chronic course – sometimes years before coming to clinical attention. In contrast to illness anxiety disorder, where patients present with anxiety about having or acquiring a serious illness in the presence of no or minimal physical symptoms, James did describe very specific symptoms which are highly associated with a panic attack based on the DSM-5 criteria. Furthermore, health concerns associated with illness anxiety disorder are incessant, even if they fluctuate and change over time, whereas James' distress about his health is largely limited to the period during, and in relation to, his unambiguous panic attacks.

Management and Treatment

The treatment for panic disorder is often twofold, including pharmacotherapy and psychotherapy. Evidence-based psychotherapy options include cognitive behavioral therapy (CBT) and psychodynamic psychotherapy. CBT is often considered first-line treatment given robust evidence available in support of this time-limited therapy, which focuses on a problem-solving approach and correction of common cognitive distortions [2]. The clinician might also consider psychodynamic psychotherapy, which promotes insight into psychological conflicts and interpersonal functioning that might contribute to the development and perpetuation of panic disorder while utilizing the therapeutic alliance [3]. Serotonin reuptake inhibitors (SRIs) are commonly the mainstay of medication treatment for panic disorder, though other types of antidepressants also have evidence for use. Benzodiazepines may be used temporarily, with caution for overuse and potential for impeding the progress of psychological therapies, such as CBT. Studies have shown that a combination of psychotherapy (CBT) and pharmacology is more effective than either treatment alone [4].

Principles for Doctors Treating Doctors

During their first session together, Dr. Waser and James carefully reviewed his symptoms and his medical work-up. James wanted to make sure to cover every possible diagnosis and potential treatment options to make sure that nothing was "overlooked." Dr. Waser thought to himself that this request

represented a kind of a "test" for James to make certain that
Dr. Waser was indeed a knowledgeable physician. However,
Dr. Waser also knew that this was at least in part the result of
James' shame and vulnerability of experiencing symptoms
that were seemingly outside of his control. It was evident,
without being explicitly stated by the patient, that James was
questioning his own ability to take care of his patients in light
of his inability to manage these symptoms and difficulties he
was having. Still not knowing much about James' life and narrative, Dr. Waser recognized that the adoption of the "patient
role" would be challenging for James. In response, Dr. Waser
highlighted James' motivation to pursue treatment as a way
to "take care of this issue" and praised his dedication to
becoming a skillful physician. It was important to emphasize
such internal strengths in order to build and reinforce James'
confidence as well as nurture their therapeutic alliance.

During the following session, Dr. Waser summarized their
previous discussion and presented James with his diagnosis of
panic disorder. Psychoeducation around the diagnosis can
help patients understand the nature of their struggles and
address any issues over self-blame or efficacy as a medical
professional. Reminding patients that there are treatments
available and prognosis is optimistic can be encouraging and
bring significant relief. As such, Dr. Waser reviewed the proposed treatments including medication and psychotherapy,
and they developed a treatment plan together. James readily
expressed interest in pursuing a time-limited focused psychotherapy such as CBT given his strong desire to rapidly "overcome and master" his symptoms. He expressed a desire to
"do this myself –without meds." Dr. Waser agreed that it
would be very reasonable to start with CBT, and delay any
decision to pharmacotherapy at this point, with the option for
a trial of medication in the future if symptoms worsened or
changed.

Dr. Waser reviewed that an essential component of CBT
for panic disorder includes "homework" assignments, which
James reluctantly accepted. James was concerned that given
his busy clinical load, he might not have enough time to

"focus on the treatment." While Dr. Waser appreciated that realistic factors, such as time limitations, did undoubtedly affect a patient's ability to commit to treatment, he also understood James' response to treatment planning as a communication indicating deeper psychological processes and needs, including some degree of largely unconscious shame and insecurity triggered by the threat of dependency (to his doctor and to therapy and medication) and its associated feelings of loss of control and self-efficacy. Such responses – though common to many – may be particularly relevant among physicians and physicians-in-training, in whom mastery of the physician-role contributes to self-esteem, and reversal of that role can lead to intense (and often generalized) self-doubt, which may be guarded against with use of resistance to treatment, among other coping strategies. Dr. Waser chose not to confront or interpret such deeper meanings, knowing that, particularly at this early stage of treatment, this sort of intervention would most likely impair the therapeutic alliance, especially given James' specific needs for validation of his sense of being competent and self-sufficient. Over time, if the opportunity arose and there was a clinical indication (e.g., resistance was continually impeding progress in treatment), Dr. Waser might find a gentle way to begin exploring these areas, with special attention to not overwhelming James' narcissistic defensive style. For now, Dr. Waser would focus on encouraging adherence with the treatment as a way for James to "get back to your fullest and optimal functioning again."

A pivotal moment during the treatment occurred after James experienced yet another panic attack prior to their fourth session together and came to treatment refusing to talk. Dr. Waser was patient and allowed James the space to process his feelings. He reminded James of the purpose of their work together, and – keeping in mind James' need to feel autonomous – encouraged James, cautiously: "I know you're motivated to get better, and I'm here to help you do that – your assistant in that process. The more we can understand about what you're noticing in yourself, the more data we'll have to put our heads together and find a solution." At that, James, who had been looking down into his lap, raised his eyes and appeared to Dr. Waser to be very briefly tearful. After a pause, he began by describing himself as a "failure" who would never be able to function as a physician. With a few very gentle encouraging prompts from Dr. Waser, James was able to further elaborate on a sense of never being able to make his father proud. Dr. Waser recalled that James had associated his first panic attack with his father's heart attack 2 years prior and right before James started medical school. Dr. Waser asked if James would describe his father as a proud man. James explained that he was a surgeon who always worked long hours and never seemed to have enough time for his family. James grew up feeling that he didn't get enough of his father's attention and assuming he must just be too "needy." He found that when he talked about his father's job, his father seemed to have more interest in him. Deciding to commit to premedical studies in college, James noticed that his father became more involved in his life – checking in about his science classes and instructing him on particular research opportunities he should find "in order to make it."

Right before James began his medical studies, his father suffered a sudden heart attack and shortly thereafter passed away. Hearing this, Dr. Waser felt momentarily stunned, realizing that while talking about James' father, James seemed to be talking about someone who was still alive. He said, "that shocked you." James became tearful. After the initial tears subsided, he explained that he figured the best thing to do would be to focus completely on his studies – "to make him proud." He felt like he barely let himself think about his father and did not cry during those initial few weeks and months. He went on to explain that when he started medical school, he felt like he had "lost some of my confidence." Despite scoring well on tests, he felt overwhelmed by the idea of mastering clinical medicine. Upon starting his medical clerkships and encountering a myriad of patients with varying diagnoses, James felt "out of place – the other students were going to become great doctors, and I'm just a fraud." Dr.

Waser allowed for a moment of quiet and then said, "and it was around that time when you started having panic attacks." James seemed to appear briefly surprised, but then calmness seemed to settle in. This was a critical session in their work together because it allowed Dr. Waser and James to explore the panic attacks as a symptom related to psychological distress, including separation and loss, and insecurity.

After this session, James became more attentive to logging his panic attacks and completing his thought records. They talked about how the homework and their sessions together were ingredients to help James become an active healer of his symptoms, not a helpless victim. In subsequent sessions, James was progressively more reflective and open, using some humor and appearing at ease. In session 7, he agreed to an exposure of running up the stairway near Dr. Waser's office and to experience a rapid heart rate. This did indeed trigger panic symptoms, though "not a full-blown attack," James said.

In the next session, he admitted to not having done his homework, and he appeared more withdrawn. Dr. Waser was able to ask him if he thought that the uncomfortable experience of having panic symptoms last week was still on his mind. James scoffed at that and said that he was just "being careful." When asked to elaborate, he explained that he was actually concerned about their doctor-patient confidentiality especially since Dr. Waser was on staff at his medical school. James inquired if Dr. Waser was going to be discussing their sessions with the medical school administration. Dr. Waser understood such concerns to be valid ones. Indeed, concerns about confidentiality and stigma within the medical community may deter medical providers, including medical students, to seek help, or may complicate engagement once they come to attention. The fear of being labeled an "impaired physician" has numerous implications for James' self-confidence and his concerns about his professional career. Nonetheless, Dr. Waser also appreciated the defensive role that James' concern about confidentiality was serving – in the setting of making progress in their therapeutic relationship and in his symptoms, with the addition of an exposure treatment that led to problematic symptoms, James was likely feeling more vulnerable. Unconscious and conscious anxieties about becoming dependent ("needy") on Dr. Waser, as well as the threat of having that protector not being able to protect him from a panic attack, were leading to shoring up of his defenses, guardedness, and a rationalization about confidentiality concerns. Dr. Waser was thoughtful in how he responded. He first reassured James that their work together would not be disclosed to the medical school administration. He added that it was his job to "support you in your efforts to get stronger." He went on to say "our ultimate goal here is for you to feel ready to be fully independent – which might mean not needing any more treatment, or might mean occasionally asking for assistance if you think it would help you take the best care of yourself that you can; in a way, it might be similar to the experience of growing up."

James was quiet at the end of that session and left without making eye contact. In the next session, however, he appeared more relaxed again. He reported that he had been reflecting on his father and realized he always had a sense that his father wanted him to be "fully adult," but James felt like his job was to figure out how to do that, himself. He wondered aloud what it would have been like to feel like his father was helping to give him "the keys to becoming a man," rather than expecting him to "just get there."

Over the next few sessions, Dr. Waser and James completed CBT for panic and talked about next steps. James expressed finding the sessions "helpful," and they agreed to continue to work together with a somewhat altered frame of exploring more aspects of James' feelings about himself and other people; Dr. Waser's tentative plan was to follow a model of largely psychodynamic technique, with more supportive and cognitive behavioral interventions as needed.

In thinking about James and their work together, Dr. Waser noticed a few themes in his countertransference. He was aware of a sense of wanting to serve as a father to James – to "fill in the deficits" that James' father, at least based on James' report, was not able to adequately do. He also noticed intermittent feelings of inefficacy and insecurity, doubting his abilities, despite his many years of experience. He understood these responses as reflecting James' own unconscious struggles with dependence vs. autonomy and power vs. weakness and vulnerability. He was able to process these responses and use them effectively to guide him in how and when to make interpretations. Very occasionally, Dr. Waser noted a desire to belittle James – moments of wondering when James would get "better." "After all," Dr. Waser would think, "we've all gone through the rigors of medical school; you just need to handle it, right?" He conceptualized these feelings as being related to identification with James as another member of the medical profession and how James' vulnerability could make Dr. Waser feel vulnerable. Overall, Dr. Waser felt a sense of satisfaction in their treatment, at times noticing a sense of intense pride. He was able to identify how some of this came from a grandiose projection from James to be considered competent and successful and his eagerness to please. He also understood this as reflecting James' more developed capacity for positive parental transference, something that Dr. Waser considered a sign of success of their treatment.

Outcome

James continued to work with Dr. Waser for the rest of the medical school, and for his first year of residency, remaining in the same institution for a transitional year before moving elsewhere in the country for a spot in the competitive field in which he had successfully matched. As they turned their attention to termination in the final year of treatment, Dr. Waser and James spent time reflecting on what James would take from the treatment and internalize. James was able to talk about how this upcoming loss would be different from the loss of his father – in that it was planned and expected and one that he felt like he might be ready for. He also noted that he felt confident in the progress he made in his life during their work together and that he believed that Dr. Waser shared that impression. They talked about next steps, including being on the watch for times and situations that might be particularly likely to contribute to recurrence of anxiety symptoms – many of which were lurking in the coming months, including a move to an unfamiliar city with few personal connections and the tasks of adapting and acculturating to the role of his chosen specialty, as well as other future points of change and insecurity. James chose not to take referrals from Dr. Waser for providers in his new city, saying he would like to "try it on my own." A month after James moved away, Dr. Waser received a phone message from James, wishing him well, saying "things are good," and asking if he might "request those referrals now, after all." Dr. Waser reflected on this communication and smiled as he thought about the rapprochement phase of development – though speculation and his sense and hope was that this was James touching base, and tolerating some need for dependency, as part of his process of taking steps forward while still feeling the support of secure attachment. Dr. Waser called James, got his voicemail, and left a message with encouraging words and the name of a colleague to call.

Pearls
- Panic disorder can present in the context of life transitions and losses. Medical school, with its frequent transitions and always-changing stressors, may be a time when a predisposed individual will experience the onset of panic disorder.
- Stigma and concerns about confidentiality of treatment and potential impact of mental health treatment on one's future career are barriers to care that commonly arise during the engagement of the trainee-patient. Addressing these concerns directly through psychoeducation can be useful; the psychia-

trist should also be considering deeper layers of meaning of these concerns as resistances to treatment and might consider interpretations if and when appropriate.

- Many medical conditions and medications or other substances can mimic panic disorder; thorough, while judicious, medical work-up and history gathering are essential to the psychiatric evaluation.

References

1. American Psychiatric Association. Diagnostic and statistical manual of mental disorders. 5th ed. Arlington: American Psychiatric Publishing; 2013.
2. Roy-Byrne PP, Craske MG, Stein MB, Sullivan G, Bystritsky A, Katon W, Sherbourne CD. A randomized effectiveness trial of cognitive-behavioral therapy and medication for primary care panic disorder. Arch Gen Psychiatry. 2005;62(3):290–8.
3. Milrod B, Chambless DL, Gallop R, Busch FN, Schwalberg M, McCarthy KS, Gross C, Sharpless BA, Leon AC, Barber JP. Psychotherapies for panic disorder: a tale of two sites. J Clin Psychiatry. 2016;77:927–35.
4. Furukawa TA, Watanabe N, Churchill R. Combined psychotherapy plus antidepressants for panic disorder with or without agoraphobia. Cochrane Database Syst Rev. 2007;(1):CD004364.

Suggested Reading

Barlow DH, Craske MG. Mastery of your anxiety and panic: workbook. 4th ed. New York: Oxford University Press; 2006.
Busch FN, Milrod BL, Sandberg LS. A study demonstrating efficacy of a psychoanalytic psychotherapy for panic disorder: implications for psychoanalytic research, theory, and practice. J Am Psychoanal Assoc. 2009;57:131–48.

Chapter 4
The Case of Ramona Williams: Losing Touch

Renee Saenger

Case

Ramona is a 26-year-old M.D.-Ph.D. candidate who presented to the emergency room late on a Sunday night. In an irritable manner she informed the emergency room psychiatrist Dr. Silva that she did not need to be evaluated, but "my husband made me come here." After a long pause and without making eye contact, she told Dr. Silva, "I guess you could say I've been anxious." Dr. Silva learned that Ramona had recently started her major clinical year after spending 3 years in the laboratory doing molecular biology research. Ramona was evasive with Dr. Silva and perseverated over her discharge from the emergency room. "It's hard to explain," she repeated when asked about her anxiety. "I'm not sure you're the right person to talk to. You look very young. Is there anyone here who is older?" Her sentences were stilted and interrupted by long pauses, but her thought process was linear. Although her husband had accompanied her to the emergency room, she refused to provide his name or phone number. Appearing scared and disheveled, Ramona

R. Saenger, MD (✉)
Weill Cornell Medical College/New York-Presbyterian Hospital-
Westchester Division, White Plains, NY, USA
e-mail: rcs7001@med.cornell.edu

© Springer Nature Switzerland AG 2019
J. S. Gordon-Elliott, A. H. Rosen (eds.), *Early Career Physician Mental Health and Wellness*,
https://doi.org/10.1007/978-3-030-10952-3_4

eventually revealed that she was also having difficulty sleeping since the beginning of her clinical rotations 2 months ago. Whereas in the laboratory her schedule had been flexible, she was now struggling to get to the hospital on time and often felt she could not keep up with the rapid pace of patient care. She no longer felt motivated to continue with the clinical rotations and felt frustrated with her husband for urging her to continue when "he doesn't understand what's going on." She had vague thoughts of returning to research, but "I had to leave the lab and I could never go back." Ramona eventually disclosed that she felt "targeted" by her former research mentor and lab colleagues. She went into great detail about each member of the lab, both male and female, and the role that each had played in a conspiracy "to bring me down and destroy the world." She looked around nervously as she spoke. On this topic Ramona became talkative and appeared animated. Ramona was certain that her home computer had been infiltrated by members of the lab. "I have very valuable data on my personal computer and they want it." Dr. Silva had to eventually end the interview because Ramona was so absorbed in her descriptions of a conspiracy. Ramona denied feeling sad or down, denied auditory or visual hallucinations, denied substance or other medication use, and denied suicidal thoughts or thoughts to harm anyone else. This was her first encounter with the mental health system.

Dr. Silva was able to find Ramona's husband in the waiting area. He described a marked change in Ramona's personality over the last year. She had become secretive and consumed with the idea that she was the target of a conspiracy involving the CIA and her research colleagues. "It's all she wants to talk about anymore…it's absurd…I miss the old Ramona." He revealed that Ramona struggled to complete her dissertation and had been reluctant to defend her thesis out of concern that "they'll take something from me," though ultimately with support from her husband managed to earn her doctorate. He brought Ramona's journal with him to the emergency room which outlined elaborate details of her fears of a joint conspiracy between her lab and the government to use her data to create genetically modified crops that would poison people. Lately she had stayed up all night writing and had gone days without eating. He observed her on several occasions carrying on heated conversations as if there were others in the room. She had also become increasingly irritable and impulsive. Last week she began to insist that they sell their house immediately because she was certain there were hidden cameras placed there by members of her lab. At times she has expressed suspiciousness toward her husband. Ramona's husband thought that Ramona's mother might have had a similar paranoid illness but did not know the exact diagnosis.

In the emergency room, Ramona accepted the recommended blood work, urine test, and brain MRI which were all unremarkable. Dr. Silva urged Ramona to accept voluntary hospitalization in order to provide diagnostic clarification and more intensive treatment. Ramona was interested in reading the voluntary hospitalization paperwork, which she pored over for almost an hour but then ultimately refused to sign in and demanded to go home. She cited her responsibilities as a medical student and alluded to her safety. "I need to get out of here." With the support of Ramona's husband, Dr. Silva made the decision to hospitalize Ramona involuntarily. Dr. Silva left a message for Ramona's faculty adviser at the medical school.

Principles of Diagnosis and Management

Diagnosis

The most appropriate diagnosis for Ramona is schizophrenia. Patients with schizophrenia exhibit a 6-month period of functional decline during which at least 1 month must include two of the following: delusions, hallucinations, disorganized speech, grossly disorganized or catatonic behavior, and negative symptoms (i.e., diminished emotional expression or avolition). Psychosis is often preceded by a prodromal period in which the presentation is primarily negative symptoms, or the psychosis is attenuated. For 1 year, Ramona's husband has been concerned for her increasing preoccupation with a conspiracy involving her lab. Her paranoid thoughts have a fixed quality highly suggestive of psychosis. Additionally, her husband has witnessed her responding to internal stimuli which are likely auditory hallucinations. Her psychotic symptoms have been accompanied by a reduced ability to perform academically as reflected in her struggle to complete her PhD. The past 2 months of clinical work have been particularly difficult due to the anxiety that often accompanies psychosis. Ramona is unable to focus and attend to the needs of her patients.

Dr. Silva's differential diagnosis for Ramona's symptoms included delusional disorder, schizoaffective disorder, bipolar disorder, major depressive disorder with psychotic features, and psychotic disorder due to another medical condition. Ramona's husband's description of his wife as staying up all night writing led Dr. Silva to consider a diagnosis of mania, but on exam Ramona did not exhibit elevated mood, pressured speech, increased energy, or disinhibited behaviors. Rather she appeared scared and seemingly unable to express herself at times. Increased talkativeness occurred only in the setting of describing her delusional system, which was a highly stimulating topic for her. Neither did Ramona report symptoms consistent with a depressed mood, which might point to a diagnosis of schizoaffective disorder if her psychotic symptoms preceded a discrete period of depression. If she were not hallucinating, she might meet criteria for delusional disorder as she remains relatively organized in her thought process. While the bloodwork, urine test, and brain imaging likely ruled out other etiologies including substance abuse and infectious or structural brain abnormalities (i.e., tumor), Dr. Silva might keep in mind that psychosis can occur in the setting of seizures and both infectious and autoimmune encephalitis.

Management and Treatment

The NICE guidelines and the American Psychiatric Association's guidelines for treatment of schizophrenia summarize the clinical management and treatment of patients with schizophrenia [1]. Patients with a "first-break" episode of psychosis should be offered both oral antipsychotic medication in conjunction with family therapy and individual cognitive behavioral therapy. The prompt initiation of treatment is recommended even before the precise diagnosis is known. Untreated and prolonged episodes of psychosis become increasingly difficult to treat. As the psychiatrist refines the diagnosis by collecting laboratory work, collateral, and historical information, it is of the utmost importance to establish a therapeutic alliance with the psychotic patient to promote adherence to care. Finally, a careful safety assessment should be completed at each patient encounter [2].

A patient like Ramona might benefit from the initiation and gradual titration of an oral antipsychotic medication. The CATIE study showed no significant difference in treatment outcomes between patients with schizophrenia treated with either typical or atypical antipsychotic medications [3]. The side effects of each class of medications and the patient's individual symptoms must be considered when choosing what medication to start. For Ramona, an atypical antipsychotic that also promotes sleep such as risperidone, olanzapine, or quetiapine might be helpful assuming that she has psychiatric follow-up in place.

Principles for Doctors Treating Doctors

Onset of schizophrenia usually occurs in the third decade for both men and women. For women, the incidence is bimodal, with increased onset in young adulthood and again postmenopause [4]. An emergency room psychiatrist like Dr. Silva is attuned to these high-risk periods and immediately suspects a psychotic process in a young woman like Ramona who is highly guarded and wary of medical evaluation. Despite Ramona's irritable demeanor and at times devaluing comments, Dr. Silva recognized that like all patients Ramona is ambivalent about receiving treatment. Ramona came willingly to the psychiatric emergency room which reflected her high level of distress. She was aware that her symptoms were not compatible with her new clinical responsibilities. Though she did not disclose these details to Dr. Silva, Ramona had already been approached by her medicine clerkship director who had been alerted by the house staff to her concerning behaviors. Ramona had not submitted patient care notes since the beginning of the rotation, was distracted during classes and in her interactions with patients, and was frequently absent without explanation. Dr. Silva did not initially ask Ramona about her interactions with the medical school administration but suspected based on her presentation that Ramona had aroused concern. Instead, Dr. Silva openly empathized with Ramona about how grueling medical training can be and wondered out loud how Ramona could be better supported. In response to her devaluing comments about her age, Dr. Silva agreed that experience is invaluable but that she was closer to Ramona's age and remembered well her own medicine rotation. Dr. Silva, a younger female attending, was cautiously trying to forge an alliance with a paranoid patient and simultaneously maintain a doctor-patient boundary. Importantly, Dr. Silva was able to recognize her countertransference toward this patient and did not respond in a confrontational or defensive manner. Ramona had learned to conceal her paranoid thoughts based on reactions from her classmates as well as her husband but did disclose her delusional thoughts to Dr. Silva which was a testament to Dr. Silva's skill. Alarmingly, Ramona appeared to have no insight surrounding her paranoid delusions. Dr. Silva felt she needed to hospitalize her involuntarily given the potential safety concerns that could arise for patients in Ramona's care.

The day after Ramona's admission to an inpatient psychiatry unit, Dr. Silva received a call from the medical clerkship director. Each medical school has its own approach to students with mental illness. Efforts have been made to reduce the stigma of mental illness, and increasing attention is being given to the higher incidence of suicide among physicians. As a psychiatrist, Dr. Silva was in a position to provide psychoeducation to nonpsychiatric medical staff. Importantly she could speak to the efficacy of antipsychotic medication and encouraged an individualized and supportive approach to Ramona's illness. The medical school, with the consent of Ramona, was in touch with Ramona's inpatient treatment team. The medical school informed her clinical supervisors that she would be absent for the remaining of the rotation to tend to her own medical needs. Ramona's treatment was a priority as was attention to her privacy as a patient receiving care.

Ramona accepted treatment with an antipsychotic during her admission and her symptoms greatly diminished. She was no longer preoccupied with her laboratory data being coveted by the government and could identify this train of thought as delusional. She wished to continue her medical training and chose to continue her psychiatric treatment as an outpatient. Her husband, also a scientist, remained her bedrock of support. Ramona agreed to meet monthly with a designated advisor from the medical school who could serve as a liaison to the administration. He was well-versed in the topic of "wellness," and appreciated that this was a critical area for Ramona as she attempted to continue her physician training. Regular sleep, exercise, healthy eating habits, and activities and relationships outside of medicine are important for all medical students but particularly for someone like Ramona with severe mental illness who was highly vulnerable to stress and sleep deprivation.

Outcome

Ramona remained adherent to outpatient psychiatric treatment. She was stabilized on an antipsychotic and engaged in cognitive behavioral therapy (CBT) for psychosis which helped her to reframe her perceptions and adjust her behavior. Ramona developed coping strategies to mitigate the perceived power of her auditory hallucinations and reduced her "appeasement" of the voices. CBT additionally helped Ramona to reality test her worries and enhance positive thoughts about herself [5]. Throughout her treatment Ramona's husband remained very involved in her care. Ramona was able to finish her medicine rotation but relapsed and had a second psychotic episode during her subsequent rotation. In total, she required hospitalization four times during the remainder of medical school. She did however successfully complete all of her rotations and was able to graduate. She decided not to participate in the residency match and instead accepted a postdoctoral position in a neuroscience laboratory where she could resume her interest in basic science and create a more flexible and manageable schedule for herself. She found it gratifying to be involved in research that could shed light on the biological underpinnings of her own mental illness.

Pearls
- Suspect a primary psychotic illness in a young adult who is exhibiting a reduced ability to function in his or her role, poor self-care, bizarre or erratic behaviors, irritability, and overt delusional thoughts and/or interaction with internal stimuli. Affective illness, substance abuse, and organic etiology must be ruled out.
- The treatment of choice for psychosis is a combination of antipsychotic medication, cognitive behavioral therapy, and family therapy. A "wellness" component that focuses on healthy lifestyle habits is particularly important given the increased risk of relapse due to sleep deprivation and stress of medical training.

- Medical schools in conjunction with treating psychiatrists can destigmatize psychotic illness by providing psychoeducation and supports to doctors and doctors-in-training.

References

1. Kuipers E, et al. Management of psychosis and schizophrenia in adults: summary of updated NICE guidance. BMJ. 2014;348:g1173. https://doi.org/10.1136/bmj.g1173.
2. Lowdermilk E, Joseph N, Feinstein RE. The treatment of schizophrenia spectrum and other psychotic disorders. In: Feinstein R, Connelly J, Feinstein M, editors. Integrating behavioral health and primary care. Oxford, UK: Oxford University Press; 2017. p. 199–223.
3. Lieberman JA, et al. Effectiveness of antipsychotic drugs in patients with chronic schizophrenia. N Engl J Med. 2005;353(12):1209–23.
4. Kirkbride JB, et al. Incidence of schizophrenia and other psychoses in England, 1950–2009: a systematic review and meta-analyses. PLoS One. 2012;7(3):e31660.
5. Lincoln TM, Peters E. A systematic review and discussion of symptom specific cognitive behavioural approaches to delusions and hallucinations. Schizophr Res. 2018. https://doi.org/10.1016/j.schres.2017.12.014.

Suggested Reading

Frese III, Frederick J, Knight EL, Saks E. Recovery from schizophrenia: with views of psychiatrists, psychologists, and others diagnosed with this disorder. Schizophr Bull. 2009;35(2):370–80.
Keshavan MS, Roberts M, Wittmann D. Guidelines for clinical treatment of early course schizophrenia. Curr Psychiatry Rep. 2006;8(4):329–34.

Chapter 5
The Case of Daniel Terzi: Trauma with Clinical Care

Rebecca Fein and Anna H. Rosen

Case

Daniel Terzi, a 26-year-old third-year medical student, presented to student health at the strong encouragement of his girlfriend for evaluation of poor sleep and decline in function over eight weeks.

While Daniel passed his pre-clerkship rotations, he did not do as well as he wanted. Specifically, he struggled with test-related anxiety. Testing was always stressful for Daniel, but this mushroomed during his first two years of medical school. Daniel was determined to perform at the top of his class during his clinical clerkships. Clinical care, he reminded himself, was the reason he wanted to become a physician. Daniel's first rotation was psychiatry. He was assigned to the acute psychotic disorders inpatient unit at a busy public hospital.

R. Fein, MD
Weill Cornell Medical College/New York-Presbyterian Hospital, New York, NY, USA
e-mail: ref9029@nyp.org

A. H. Rosen, MD (✉)
Weill Cornell Medical College/New York-Presbyterian Hospital-Westchester Division, White Plains, NY, USA
e-mail: ash9006@med.cornell.edu

© Springer Nature Switzerland AG 2019   45
J. S. Gordon-Elliott, A. H. Rosen (eds.), *Early Career Physician Mental Health and Wellness*,
https://doi.org/10.1007/978-3-030-10952-3_5

He was excited about his assignment and within his first week, already felt part of a team treating challenging and interesting patients.

At the start of the second week of this rotation, Daniel began working with Mr. L, a 40-year-old man with schizophrenia. Mr. L was admitted over the weekend following an unprovoked verbal altercation with a group of women on the street. Since his presentation to the emergency room, Mr. L was noted to be paranoid and irritable. He refused all medications, but considering his disorganization and agitation, he required emergency intramuscular medications and restraints on multiple occasions. The attendings on Daniel's unit emphasized that the experience for psychotic patients was scary and the level of their paranoia could provoke unpredictable and aggressive behaviors. Medications were part of his treatment.

Mr. L's treatment team knew that he required ongoing neuroleptic medications to treat his psychosis and address his associated dangerousness. He continued to refuse medications, and his treatment team began legal proceedings for treatment over objection. The day before Mr. L was to go to court, Daniel met with Mr. L in his room and attempted to persuade Mr. L to take medications without involving the legal system. He believed that they had developed a nice rapport seeing each other during rounds every day and nodding hello to each other regularly on the inpatient unit. Daniel imagined that approaching Mr. L individually in his room, Mr. L would feel less scared. On approach, Mr. L was initially calm, but as Daniel broached the topic of medication, Mr. L's behavior shifted and became threatening. Daniel started to leave Mr. L's room when Mr. L lunged at him, knocking him to the ground with a punch to his nose. Daniel raced out of Mr. L's room and left the unit without any staff witnessing the aftermath of a bloody nose. Daniel went home and reached out to his attending to say that he had "food poisoning" and would be back at work the following day.

Daniel was primarily concerned that his decision to meet alone with Mr. L and Mr. L's aggression reflected his futility as a health-care provider. He believed he would fail the clerkship and perhaps face disciplinary action. Daniel did not inform his attending nor did he report the incident to the medical school; instead, he continued to work on the unit as a member of Mr. L's treatment team. Following the incident, Daniel started to have significant trouble sleeping, with frequent nightmares that woke him from sleep with accompanying palpitations and the image of Mr. L knocking him to the ground. It was difficult for him to concentrate in both social and academic settings. Furthermore, he was anxious when he attempted to do required readings and on edge when asked to present during rounds. In fact, he had called out sick multiple times over subsequent weeks, as he felt significantly more uncomfortable when in the hospital building. Daniel's girlfriend was concerned about his low mood, lack of interest in doing activities together, and overall decline in functioning. She finally insisted that he seek psychiatric evaluation after he became furious with her when she accidently startled him while they were studying together in the library.

Daniel insisted that his girlfriend accompany him to his initial evaluation at student health where he met with a psychiatrist, Dr. Mada, a recent graduate of his medical school's psychiatry residency program. Daniel was scared. He scanned Dr. Mada's office throughout the session. He was reluctant to talk about the assault and focused on his poor sleep as a result of his recurrent nightmares.

Principles of Diagnosis and Management

Diagnosis

Daniel presented to student health with symptoms of anxiety that started after a potentially fatal experience. This traumatic experience prompted the re-experiencing of the event via nightmares, as well as hypervigilance, with poor concentration, difficulty sleeping, and increased startle response. The most appropriate diagnosis for Daniel is post-traumatic stress disorder (PTSD) [see Table 5.1]. Patients with PTSD have experienced or witnessed a traumatic event that is life-threatening or potentially life-threatening in nature. Following such a catastrophic trauma, such individuals experience intrusive symptoms including unwanted memories, flashbacks, emotional distress or physical reactivity when reminded of the traumatic event. Individuals may also demonstrate avoidance behavior which can include avoidance of trauma-related stimuli [1]. As exhibited in Daniel's case, PTSD can also impact one's mood and inhibit their daily functioning. While Daniel meets criteria for PTSD, other possible diagnoses should be considered. Adjustment disorder with anxious features is on the differential; however, such a diagnosis typically applies to stressful life events that are not life-threatening in nature. In the case of Daniel's physical assault, his life was, in fact, threatened. Another possible diagnosis is major depressive disorder (MDD). Daniel's poor sleep, diminished concentration, and low mood over a period greater than 2 weeks are suggestive of MDD; however, in order to firmly make this diagnosis, more information about recent symptoms is necessary. Given Daniel's current level of hyperarousal and anxiety

TABLE 5.1 Post-traumatic stress disorder: core features

Exposure to a traumatic experience involving threat to one's life or safety (physical or sexual), through direct exposure, witnessing, on behalf of a loved one, or in a recurrent way
At least 1 month of:
Intrusion symptoms related to the trauma (e.g., memories, dreams, dissociative symptoms, or other distressing emotional or physical symptoms)
Avoidance of thoughts or cues related to the trauma
Problematic changes in thinking or emotions (e.g., altered memory of the event, negative thoughts about oneself, low mood)
Changes in arousal and behavior (e.g., irritability, recklessness, heightened attention, impaired sleep)

(with associated difficulty concentration and sleep disturbances), combined with his previous history of anxiety during pre-clerkship years, an anxiety disorder should also be considered. In order to make this diagnosis, more information would have to be obtained about the nature of his anxieties beyond that related to traumatic event. A diagnosis of complex PTSD should also be considered. This is relevant for patients concurrently experiencing emotional dissociation, emotion deregulation, somatization, and strained relationships. Daniel's symptoms have persisted for over a month following the event, and as such, acute stress disorder is not on the differential, which is a transient state and passes within one month. Furthermore, the possible role of alcohol and other substances should be considered as a possible diagnosis. While his case presentation does not specifically reference signs or symptoms that are directly suggestive of substance use, his rather sudden change of behavior could be explained by acute intoxication and/or withdrawal.

Management and Treatment

PTSD diagnosis and treatment begin with a thorough evaluation. Treatment options include psychopharmacologic management and/or psychotherapy. This decision is largely based on patient's individual preference and treatment availability. If medication is indicated, antidepressants, usually serotonin reuptake inhibitors (SRIs), are prescribed. SRIs can help a patient feel less on edge, decrease irritability, and help lift one's mood. In addition to antidepressant medications, other classes of medications, such as benzodiazepines (fast-acting anxiolytics) to target moments of panic and hypervigilance, are beneficial when use cautiously and judiciously. Alpha-1 adrenergic receptor blockers (to address nightmares) can also be considered as augmentation agents. Psychotherapy can be used in place of, or in addition to, medications. Possible therapy modalities to consider include trauma-based therapy, cognitive behavioral therapy, eye movement desensitization and reprocessing (EMDR), or supportive psychotherapy [2]. Previous studies have shown that trauma-focused psychotherapies can help decrease the severit of one's symptoms. For example, a meta-analysis found that trauma-focused cognitive behavior therapy led to greater reduction in PTSD symptoms than usual care [3]. In individuals such as Daniel, therapy can play a crucial role in addressing ongoing symptoms while also promoting coping skills necessary to tolerate future distressing circumstances.

Principles for Doctors Treating Doctors

Upon initial presentation to Dr. Mada, Daniel expressed ambivalence about receiving psychiatric care. On the one hand, he recognized the recent changes in his level of functioning, subsequently negatively impacting his academic performance and relationship with his girlfriend. That said, he was preoccupied that seeking mental health treatment would influence his standing in medical school. Daniel was concerned he would be penalized not only for his clinical judgment prior to the assault but also because he could not control his symptoms. It was also very uncomfortable to recount the details of the event. He wondered if others would fear him as a psychiatric patient in the way others perceived Mr. L on the inpatient unit. In fact, Daniel's fear of stigma played a large role in his decision not to tell supervisors about the assault when it occurred. Daniel shared the events with Dr. Mada as well as the changes he noticed about himeslf over the last two months. His major concern was difficulty sleeping, as he awoke from nightmares multiple times per night. Lack of sleep was leading to exhaustion during the day and decline in his academic performance. Furthermore, he was having a substantial level of anxiety when in the hospital for required hospital rotations; he shared that he recently had to leave a patient's room during rounds, as a patient suddenly moved in his bed to reach for his cell phone, leaving Daniel sweaty, breathing quickly, and panicky. Daniel was unsure how he would continue with his clerkships.

Dr. Mada proceeded with a comprehensive review of symptoms, including substance use, mood symptoms, psychotic symptoms, and suicidality, as PTSD is often associated with high rates of psychiatric comorbidities [4]. Daniel denied symptoms concerning for an additional condition. Dr. Mada diagnosed Daniel with PTSD related to his assault. While Daniel acknowledged he was "stressed," he did not agree that he met diagnostic criteria for such a serious mental illness. He was also concerned that the details of the event would travel from Dr. Mada to the inpatient psychiatry attending on the unit. Dr. Mada emphasized the benefits of beginning treatment right away in order to avoiding long-standing impairments. He recommended initiating both medication and therapy. Daniel was hesitant to commit to treatment, especially weekly therapy, as he felt like his busy academic schedule precluded him from such intensive care. Dr. Mada impressed upon Daniel that addressing his well-being was an essential element of professionalism. He needed to care for himself in order to care for others. Ultimately, Daniel agreed to begin a medication trial. Escitalopram, a selective serotonin reuptake inhibitor (SSRI), was started at a low dose and subsequently increased to the higher end of therapeutic doses. Daniel noted some improvement in his baseline level of anxiety and isolation but continued to experience sleep disturbances and hypervigilance, especially when in the hospital setting. In addition to the escitalopram, Dr. Mada recommended Daniel to take prazosin at bedtime to target ongoing nightmares and sleep disturbances [5]. While on this medication regimen, Daniel had a partial response but continued to have difficulty spending time alone with patients. He agreed to augment medications with trauma-focused cognitive behavioral therapy.

Dr. Mada referred Daniel to a therapist, Dr. Guy, who was trained specifically in trauma-focused cognitive behavioral therapy (TF-CBT) [6]. The goal of TF-CBT is to help individuals reconceptualize their traumatic experiences, their capacity for resilience and the ability to cope following the trauma [7]. Daniel had weekly individual sessions, where he was encouraged to re-evaluate his automatic thoughts about the assault that were often catastrophic and negative in nature. He was asked to participate in a range of different exposure activities that directly addressed his avoidance behaviors. For example, in order to challenge anxieties related to spending time in the hospital, and specifically alone with patients, Daniel composed a graded exposure hierarchy in which he was alone with patients across a variety of settings. During such exposures, his therapist asked him to keep detailed thought records, where he identified automatic thoughts, as well as associated emotions, adaptive responses, and outcome to exposures. As part of Daniel's exposure heirarchy, Daniel reached out to his inpatient attending to discuss the event. Reflecting on this exposure with Dr. Guy, Daniel reconceptualized his experience on the inpatient unit as a wish to appear capable as a medical student and empathic as a provider to Mr. L. Because his intervention with Mr. L, did not go as planned he felt shame and this inhibited him from reaching out for supervision at the time of the episode. This was one example of reconceptualizing his experience and understanding alternative ways of coping with the trauma. With ongoing therapy, Daniel challenged his thinking patterns related to patient care and the possibility of a subsequent assault. He focused on building skills to tolerate patient encounters and time in the hospital.

Outcome

Daniel continued to work with both Dr. Mada for medication management and Dr. Guy for therapy. He was maintained on escitalopram 20 mg daily to target anxiety. Prazosin was tapered off over subsequent months, as his sleep improved. After completing the course of trauma-focused cognitive behavioral therapy, Daniel continued to meet with Dr. Guy weekly, but the focus of therapy shifted to more supportive and dynamic in nature. Goals included addressing Daniel's baseline anxiety and develop a better understanding why he did not disclose the assault or associated difficulties to his medical school administration. Specific emphasis was placed on exploring his tendency to avoid asking for support from others, given the concern that doing so would make him seem less capable or intelligent. Over the following year, Daniel gained insight into his perfectionistic tendencies and desire to present himself as infallible regardless of the circumstances. He was able to reflect on the fact that the unrealistic expectations he was placing on himself led to anxiety that was inhibiting his ability to succeed. Daniel was able to complete all of his clerkships and is now preparing to apply for a position in a pediatrics residency program.

Pearls

- Post-traumatic stress disorder (PTSD) is a psychiatric condition that can affect any individual exposed to a trauma that involves an actual or threatened injury to oneself or others. Symptoms include intrusive thoughts, nightmares, and flashbacks, as well as hypervigilance, avoidance of reminders of the trauma, and sleep disturbance.
- Psychiatric comorbidity is high in individuals with PTSD, and therefore careful attention must be paid to evaluating for comorbid mood disorders, anxiety disorders, and substance use disorders.
- PTSD is best managed when treatment begins as quickly as possible after a person is diagnosed with this condition; that being said, many individuals are resistant to receiving care.
- Treatment of PTSD can include medications and psychotherapy. These two approaches can be used individually or in conjunction with each other. Deciding which modality to begin with depends on the specifics of the individual case (i.e., patient's preference, availability of therapy, severity of symptoms).
- If an individual participates in therapy, attention should be paid to targeting symptoms specific to

PTSD but also to gaining better insight of other comorbid psychiatric conditions. Such an approach can help an individual understand underlying difficulties that contributed to the development of PTSD; with such an improved understanding, it is hopeful that the patient can enhance overall functioning and resilience in the future.

References

1. American Psychiatric Association. Diagnostic and statistical manual of mental disorders. 5th ed. Arlington: American Psychiatric Publishing; 2013.
2. Courtois CA, Sonis J, Fairbank JA, Friedman M, Jones R, Roberts J, Schulz P. Clinical practice guideline for the treatment of posttraumatic stress disorder (PTSD) in adults. American Psychological Association. 2017.
3. Bisson J, Andrew M. Psychological treatment of post-traumatic stress disorder (PTSD). Cochrane Database Syst Rev. 2007;(3):CD003388.
4. Goldstein RB, Smith SM, Chou SP, et al. The epidemiology of DSM-5 posttraumatic stress disorder in the United States: results from the national epidemiologic survey on alcohol and related conditions-III. Soc Psychiatry Psychiatr Epidemiol. 2016;51:1137.
5. Raskind MA, Peskind ER, Chow B, et al. Trial of prazosin for post-traumatic stress disorder in military veterans. N Engl J Med. 2018;378:507–17.
6. Kar N. Cognitive behavioral therapy for the treatment of post-traumatic stress disorder: a review. Neuropsychiatr Dis Treat. 2011;7:167–81.
7. Stein DJ, Ipser JC, Seedat S. Pharmacotherapy for posttraumatic stress disorder (PTSD). Cochrane Database Syst Rev. 2006;(1):CD002795.

Suggested Reading

Goodnight JRM, Ragsdale KA, Rauch SAM, Rothbaum BO. Psychotherapy for PTSD: an evidence-based guide to a theranostic approach to treatment. Prog Neuro-Psychopharmacol Biol Psychiatry. 2019;88:418.

Zoellner LA, Roy-Byrne PP, Mavissakalian M, Feeny NC. Doubly randomized preference trial of prolonged exposure versus sertraline for treatment of PTSD. Am J Psychiatr. 2018.

Chapter 6
The Case of Abigail Nunce: The Weight of Medical Training

Janna S. Gordon-Elliott

Case

Abigail Nunce is a 25-year-old third year medical student presenting to Dr. Balan, a student mental health psychiatrist at her medical school, with a chief complaint of "I guess they're worried about my weight again, but I think I'm ok." Abigail had been referred to Dr. Balan at the request of the student health service for assessment of an eating disorder in the context of her visit to the clinic with palpitations. Abigail tells Dr. Balan that she has a history of anorexia nervosa, with food restriction and weight loss at age 14, which improved over the next 2 years with individual and family therapy and nutritional counseling. She states that she had been "fine – that is all behind me," but during the course of studying for her STEP-1 exam, just before starting her first clerkship, she noticed that some of her old preoccupations with her food intake and weight had started to "crop up" again. She reports that after a couple of years of rarely getting on the scale, she

J. S. Gordon-Elliott, MD (✉)
Weill Cornell Medical College/New York-Presbyterian Hospital,
New York, NY, USA
e-mail: jsg2005@med.cornell.edu

© Springer Nature Switzerland AG 2019
J. S. Gordon-Elliott, A. H. Rosen (eds.), *Early Career Physician Mental Health and Wellness*,
https://doi.org/10.1007/978-3-030-10952-3_6

57

began weighing herself in the morning, which then became a daily habit, scrutinizing any increase or decrease by a fraction of a pound. She would pack her food for the day before going to the library to study, and she would only eat a set times, initially feeling like it was a good way of structuring the day of studying. She gradually started reducing the amount of food she was putting into her lunch and snack, and she would wait for the next morning to weigh herself to ensure her weight had gone down again, which it was doing most days – with anxiety when the number on the scale would increase by 0.2 lbs., wondering how that could be possible given that she had not eaten even "a calorie more" than the day before. She reports that she would eat exactly the same thing every day – not atypical for her, she notes – and would get nervous if a social event arose, such as dinner out with friends or (especially) an unplanned invitation for lunch with a friend she might see in the library.

After STEP-1, surgery was her first clerkship. She brought in her lunch and some snacks to make sure she ate. She found the long days challenging, as she couldn't anticipate when she could eat or when she would get home, but she found herself excited by the stimulation and activity. At the end of her first week, she felt nauseated and light-headed in her first case of the day and had to leave the operating room (OR) briefly – an incident that she found deeply humiliating, "as if I weren't tough enough to cut it." She later attributed her symptoms to having eaten her breakfast only an hour before coming into the "chemical environment" of the OR. The next day, she scrubbed into a late case which ended up going for 8 hours. Feeling energized when it finished, despite the late hour and having not eaten since that morning, she noticed a familiar feeling of "emptiness and lightness" that felt exciting – one she had experienced frequently when she would restrict in her early teens. She stopped packing lunches and began carrying a granola bar for snacking over the day, eating a small bite here and there. At the end of the clerkship, her parents had come to visit her for a week and commented on her weight loss. She reports her weight had gone down 13 pounds over the 4 months since they had seen her last, now weighing 105lbs at 5′4″ (body mass index 18.0; normal range 18.5–24.9). During the first week of her next clerkship, she had a run of heart palpitations one morning and became acutely frightened, having spent her last week on the cardiothoracic service and thinking that perhaps she had a cardiomyopathy or other cardiac issue due to her history of an eating disorder years ago. She called her mother immediately, as she often would do when she had a health concern, and her mother told her to go to student health; in the background of the call, she heard her father saying, "she hasn't been eating, she's doing it again." Feeling angry, but scared, she went to the clinic and was evaluated; her medical work-up was unremarkable, with normal labs and a normal EKG. They planned for a follow-up in 2 weeks to discuss if any further evaluation was needed; in the meantime, the student health physician suggested that she go see Dr. Balan because of the information she blurted out anxiously about her history of an eating disorder, her recent food restriction, and her fears "maybe I've really hurt myself."

In response to Dr. Balan's further questioning, Abigail admits to always having been concerned about her appearance and weight. She had gained weight in puberty and was told that her weight was "in the upper percentiles"; she thinks her food restriction followed this. Having maintained a steady weight for the past several years, she reports feeling "better" at this currently lower weight – "I just feel more comfortable." She denies any binge eating or inappropriate compensatory behaviors for weight loss, including vomiting, laxative use, or excessive exercise. She reports always having had daily rituals, including her pre-bed routine, involving several steps, taking about 15–20 minutes per evening. She denies any current alcohol use or other substance use. She is on no medications and denies taking any supplements.

Principles of Diagnosis and Management

Diagnosis

The preferred DSM-5 diagnosis for Abigail is other specified feeding or eating disorder (OSFED; anorexia nervosa, restricting type, in remission, now with symptom recurrence, not yet meeting full criteria).

Abigail has a history of anorexia nervosa (AN) as a teenager. A diagnosis of AN is made in individuals who demonstrate restricted food intake associated with significantly low body weight, intense fear of gaining weight or behavior that interferes with appropriate weight maintenance, and distorted degree to which self-esteem depends on body weight. Most likely, Abigail's current symptoms reflect reemergence of AN, given her progressive preoccupation with food intake and weight, and its connection with her self-esteem. She has lost some weight but arguably not substantial enough to meet full criteria for AN, though the criteria are loose in terms of interpretation of the amount of weight loss – a factor that can be up to clinician discretion based on the entire picture of symptomatology and severity of the situation.

As detailed below, the differential diagnosis should include consideration, and further assessment if indicated, of one of the other feeding and eating disorders (FEDs), as well as, and in addition to, other psychiatric disorders, such as anxiety, substance use, personality, and obsessive compulsive and related disorders.

Considering the other FEDs, without binge eating or compensatory behaviors, such as vomiting after eating, neither bulimia nervosa (BN) nor binge eating disorder (BED) would fit her symptoms. If she were purging occasionally but maintaining very low weight and obstructing efforts to gain weight, the appropriate diagnosis would be AN, binge-eating/purging type, not BN. Avoidant restrictive food intake disorder (ARFID), a diagnosis that was somewhat modified and recategorized in the development of DSM-5, should be considered. ARFID involves a pattern of food restriction in the absence of evidence for specific concerns about body weight. It may be diagnosed in individuals who are specifically avoiding certain foods due to features of the food (e.g., texture, color, or taste) or in some cases due to fears about the consequences of eating (such as a fear of choking), resulting in weight loss and nutritional impairment. Abigail described an episode of fearing fainting or vomiting in the OR, which she associated with eating soon before being in the room. Further probing would be appropriate to assess for whether she has more substantial concerns about a physical problem related to certain food items or having food in her stomach. In such cases, an individual might begin avoiding food/food items and lose weight; the difference with ARFID is that the intention is not to lose weight but to avoid some aversive consequence of the food (an event, an unpleasant sensation, etc.). Much less is known about ARFID in terms of prevalence in general and clinical populations, risk factors, outcomes, and treatment than about AN, BN, and BED, given a limited literature on the disorder to date. Given the clear association between Abigail's behaviors and her thoughts about her body weight and shape, ARFID would not be an appropriate diagnosis. Beyond the formal FED diagnoses, many individuals have eating symptoms that may exist for years but do not meet full criteria for one of the FEDs. Patterns of disordered eating, including frequent dieting, and significant concerns about calorie intake and weight are highly prevalent and may or may not cause distress and meet clinical attention. For example, studies have shown that up to 90% of college-aged women in the USA have dieted at some point, and the same percent of all women in the USA have some degree of body dissatisfaction [1]. Pervasive cultural ideals favoring thinness, notably in Western countries, as well as other societal pressures and mixed messages, including the ever-available presence of food juxtaposed with the inescapable weight loss industry, all contribute to a high degree of attention paid by men and women to their bodies, with resultant focus and manipulation of food intake and calorie balance.

Beyond the FEDs, Dr. Balan should be considering other diagnoses, either ones that could explain the presentation or be co-occurring with a FED. Abigail describes a highly routinized life with anxiety about disruption of her order. OCD symptoms should be further explored; obsessional thoughts or rituals should not be dual coded as OCD in a patient with a FED if these symptoms are specifically centered on food or weight. Patients with body dysmorphic disorder (BDD) have preoccupations with certain body parts and can be confused with the body image concerns of a patient with an FED; however, in BDD, the focus should be on the appearance of a particular body part, not general weight. Obsessive-compulsive personality disorder (OCPD) includes traits that can often co-occur in patients with AN, or which can be exacerbated in the setting of AN, such as intense focus on routine, order, and need for control of eating and related behaviors (such as exercise). A personality disorder diagnosis should be considered if there is adequate evidence to support significant symptoms that have existed in a consistent manner over the individual's adult life and that are causing significant distress or impairment. Many medical students, indeed, have some traits of OCPD (e.g., conscientiousness, perfectionism, some difficulty with delegating work, and a preference for structure and routine). In fact, such symptoms, when mild and somewhat flexible, may actually be adaptive for the medical professional and associated with success. When the symptoms become more pervasive and rigid, causing problems professionally or interpersonally, a personality disorder diagnosis should be considered and addressed. Anxiety disorders, such as generalized anxiety disorder or social anxiety disorder, can co-occur with FEDs and should be screened for. Substance use disorders should similarly be on the differential and reviewed.

Management and Treatment

Feeding and eating disorders commonly onset during adolescence and early adulthood, and subclinical disordered eating may be highest during this period as well, making the medical student population one in which eating issues can be routinely found. Screening for eating symptoms should be considered in the evaluation of student-patients. Short, clinician-administered screening tools include the eating disorder screen for primary care (ESP) and the SCOFF [2, 3].

Once an eating disorder, or problematic disordered eating, has been identified, the clinician will want to discuss this with the patient and assess the patient's insight and willingness for treatment. Insight can be poor in some individuals, and while the symptoms can bring great distress, they may feel ego-syntonic for the patient or the idea of losing the symptoms may feel to frightening. A motivational interviewing approach may be useful in engaging the patient's participation in treatment. When medical or psychiatric safety is at risk, further steps may be needed to begin treatment even if the patient is not willing.

All treatment planning in AN must start with a medical evaluation to establish medical stability. For those with unstable electrolytes (e.g., low potassium or sodium), severely low weight, or significant cardiac issues (extreme bradycardia or any arrhythmias), inpatient medical hospitalization may first be necessary for stabilization and cautious feeding while monitoring for refeeding syndrome. The safety evaluation must also include assessment for suicidality and self-injurious behavior (including notably, compensatory behaviors being used for weight loss, including vomiting, diuretic and laxative overuse, and extreme exercise). All in all, rates of premature death are highest in patients with AN than in any other psychiatric disorder, with mortality driven by both the medical consequences of the illness and suicide. Inpatient psychiatric hospitalization may be required when patients cannot commit to adequate engagement with outpatient treatment and are continuing to maintain a dangerously low weight or are still losing weight. Day programs developed for eating disorders can be very useful bridges to avoid or step down from inpatient hospitalization.

Maudsley family therapy is an evidence-based approach to AN for individuals who are still in their primary family unit [4], such as adolescents. This treatment engages the family in normalizing eating behavior and minimizing problematic dynamics that perpetuate the symptoms. Individual and group therapy for patients with AN commonly includes basic psychoeducation and a cognitive behavioral therapy approach in which patients learn about the cyclic association between their food restriction, weight loss, and self-esteem that leads to further food restriction, with no clear end point. Nutritional counseling is essential. Eating must be normalized, and this is may be accomplished through eating together in the group setting, keeping food logs, and progressively expanding food choices and eating flexibility over time.

At very low weight, there is no evidence that antidepressants, such as selective serotonin reuptake inhibitors (SSRIs), are effective for improving symptoms of AN. This may be related to the severe state of nutritional deficiency. There is emerging evidence for the use of atypical antipsychotics to ease anxiety related to normalizing food intake [5]. When weight begins to normalize, SSRIs may be useful for managing co-occurring syndromes of anxiety or depression that may perpetuate dependence on the eating symptoms for emotional self-management.

Principles for Doctors Treating Doctors

Dr. Balan is a general adult psychiatrist, without specific training in FEDs. Despite this, he will need to explore Abigail's symptoms with her, and if he has significant concerns for a reemergence of her AN, share that with her and engage her interest in getting the appropriate help to minimize the severity of the relapse and protect against future recurrences. With additional resources at his and Abigail's disposal, Dr. Balan can initiate a treatment team, based on Abigail's current medical, psychiatric, and interpersonal needs.

After a full history, Dr. Balan reflects back to Abigail what he has heard – a history of AN, and increasing focus on food, and progressive food restriction and weight loss in the setting of new and chronic stressors. He then asks Abigail what she thinks is going on. She sits back and is quiet for a minute, looking down at her hands. She says that the past few months "have been tough." She describes the isolation she felt during STEP-1 studying and her sense of the loss of "everything that felt normal – it was just me, studying, nothing but my own structure." She went on to say that during surgery clerkship, she felt optimistic again and connected with others but increasingly overwhelmed by the pressures of performing. She reflects that this reminded her of how she felt at the beginning of high school, just as her eating disorder was starting. She transitioned into a bigger school, with stronger "competition" and "bigger stakes." She recalls how her food restriction seemed to serve many purposes – she lost some weight, which initially was very satisfying for her, as she had been self-conscious about having "a few extra pounds on me"; she felt "strangely energized, like I could do things others couldn't – I could survive on fewer calories"; and she experienced the focus on food as "organizing," with her small meals marking out milestones of the day to "get through." She remembers also, however, becoming progressively "sad and alone." She tells Dr. Balan that she realizes this is how she feels now. She is not sure how to get better or feel better – "I don't think I can keep this up, and I don't want to give up and gain weight; I don't feel like I have options."

In response, Dr. Balan offers validation for Abigail's sense of being trapped and afraid. He reflects to her that he considers this a relapse of her AN and that he will help her find her bearings so she can climb out of this hole without it feeling too frightening. He considers, and shares with Abigail, a stress-diathesis perspective. Psychiatric disorders and symptoms may fluctuate substantially based on the experiences the individual is facing at any given time. Abigail may have a predisposition for an eating disorder based on genetic and environmental factors earlier in life, and – in her case – her past episodes. Subsequent relapses may occur in the setting of specific triggers or general overwhelming stress. It is important for the provider treating medical students to be thinking about the common stressors that face this population, and the junctures or transition points that are inherently more challenging, and which may unveil new behavioral health symptoms or lead to recurrence of previous ones. Such phases may include the very start of medical school, the beginning of the clinical years, the exam study periods (i.e., "the boards"), the residency matching period, and the end of school while the student is mentally beginning the transition to the next stage (for most, residency). Different periods of the medical school trajectory can strain individuals in varying ways. For the student with an eating disorder, a period of high stress where there is also control over one's time (such as during exam studying), having time to meal-plan may be useful in avoiding problematic symptoms, from restrictrion, to overeating, to binge-purging; whereas, the absence of external structure may, for some, lead to worsening of any of these symptoms. Similarly, a time of high stress and limited control over one's schedule, such as during clerkships, may be useful for some who find that engagement in meaningful activity and socialization helps loosen some of the obsessional thinking and lessen the pull towards symptomatic behavior, while it may be more challenging for others, especially early on during treatment, when normalization of eating patterns is an essential focus of the treatment. The clinician working with these patients should be anticipating such transitions and how they will impact the individual, specifically. In addition, it is important for the clinician to explicitly engage the student-patient to learn to be ready for these junctures and to increase self-care practices or otherwise modify lifestyle and treatment in advance in order to minimize risk during these critical times. Ultimately, a goal of treatment will be to help the student with an eating disorder to learn more tolerance for stress and ways to dissipate it and embrace it that involve more adaptive behaviors than the eating symptoms.

In beginning their treatment planning, Dr. Balan and Abigail talk about the family therapy that was prescribed for her at age 14. Once adults have separated and are no longer living with their parents, such an approach may no longer be as relevant or helpful, at least when there are fewer active dependency needs and interactions around eating on a daily basis. At age 25, Abigail is, for all intents and purposes, an adult. Many factors, nonetheless, influence the extent to which those in early adulthood have established a fully adult identity. Societal norms in the USA and similar nations have changed for social, cultural, and economic reasons, with an extension of adolescence to older ages, in which parents may not only continue to financially supplement or support their children well into their 20s but also maintain a level of personal support and oversight similar to what would be seen in the relationship between a parent and a child still living in the home. So-called "emerging adults" in their early and mid-20s may still be depending on their parents for education and housing expenses and for emotional and developmental purposes – such as frequent check-ins for guidance and supervision regarding their social, occupational, and health needs. Like many of her peers, Abigail's parents are paying for medical school, including housing; moreover, as she tells Dr. Balan, their relationship has always been one in which she looks to them for help and reassurance about many of her decisions on a regular basis. And while she lives apart from them, she reports that her mother still checks in by text three times a day to ask about her eating – a behavior that has increased in intensity recently in the setting of her parents' awareness that her symptoms may be escalating again. Dr. Balan will need to keep all of this in mind when considering his treatment recommendations with Abigail. He will want to explore with her the relationship with her parents and the extent to which that relationship might be used to help her in her treatment or the ways in which involving them could complicate or interfere with her recovery.

After his full assessment and review of her mental health and medical needs, Dr. Balan suggested to Abigail that she begin to see a therapist in the community with expertise in working with patients with eating disorders and anxiety. Abigail was reluctant but agreed to try. He also made a referral to a nutritionist with experience with eating disorders, and he let Abigail know that he would want to have an open line of communication between "the whole team," including himself, Abigail, the nutritionist, the therapist, and the student health physician. Abigail and Dr. Balan discussed medication. Abigail is underweight, but not extremely so, and she is medically stable. She is describing low mood and anxiety. They talk about the option of starting an SSRI for depression or anxiety "in a few weeks if things aren't looking up," as treating a co-occurring depressive or anxiety disorder at her current weight might help her engage more in her eating disorder treatment. Abigail acknowledges that she probably will need to loosen up on her restrictions and gain some weight – "right now, it just has too much of a hold on me" – but she says she's worried about weight gain, especially from medications. Dr. Balan states that he does not intend to give her medications just for the purpose of weight gain and that he will be thoughtful about the potential weight effects of any medication they start; ideally, through her treatment, she will gradually improve her eating and make modest weight gains on her own accord, with or without medication. Abigail expresses feeling more hope and a sense that things could "get easier."

Throughout his work with Abigail, Dr. Balan has attended to his feelings and countertransference experiences. The patient with an eating disorder can elicit a range of emotional responses in providers – from anger or frustration that can arise from the sense that the symptoms are "self-induced" to an experience of being manipulated by the patient who might be holding "secrets" about her behavior (out of concern about those behaviors being "taken away" if someone finds out, or out of *shame* – an essential feature of eating disorders and so many psychiatric disorders). Some providers may feel protective of the individual, sharing the patient's projected sense of her vulnerability and taking on the role of parent or savior. A thread that is often present in patients with AN is a juxtaposition of this vulnerability with invincibility or transcendence from the usual "rules" that all humans have to follow (i.e., eating enough calories to live). The patient may continually waver from one side to the other of this division, and the provider's countertransference responses will thusly vary. Being aware of the projections that arise, being mindful not to engage in maladaptive enactments (such as overprotection and collusion with the patient's symptoms, or punitive reactions), and maintaining empathy for the pain that the patient is feeling will be crucial for the provider. Working with a team of other providers, monitoring each other's countertransference responses, and having support for processing uncomfortable feelings that may arise during treatment, can help serve this overall purpose and help move the patient toward recovery. The psychiatrist treating a medical student may have additional responses specific to the identification with a medical trainee, including, among others, feelings of resentment that the student is "weak" and can't withstand the stressors of medical training, or desires to guard the student against "the pressures that I withstood," in so doing maintaining her dependence on the provider and perhaps, in turn, her symptoms.

Outcome

Abigail works closely with her therapist and nutritionist over the next few months to work in new foods and more flexibility around eating. She and Dr. Balan decide to try low-dose sertraline for anxiety symptoms she continues to have, and she notices a small – but tolerable – lessening of her preoccupation with food and a general relief that comes with this. She talks about exercise and how to engage in it in a healthy way without focusing too much on it as a calorie burner. She had enjoyed, and exceled in, team sports during high school, and she decided to join an adult recreational soccer league, giving her more opportunity for socialization and even the additional challenge to her rules and restrictions of going to drinks with teammates after matches.

Dr. Balan considers whether he needs to open up a discussion with medical school administration about accommodations during Abigail's upcoming clerkships, as she has, coincidentally, been in a scheduled three-month research block during this period of treatment. He and Abigail talk about this – the strain that reentry to clerkships will pose for her, with the potential to exacerbate her symptoms, as well as the ways in which she might be able to utilize the stressor of clerkships to her benefit; the has learned skills and improved in her symptoms since her surgery clerkship, and she could approach this one differently. She and the nutritionist come up with a plan for ensuring adequate eating while on clerkships, even on busy days. In her CBT, she and her therapist speak about finding ways to use the unpredictability of the clerkship as a challenge, as part of her overall goal to desensitize herself to the anxiety of having to eat more flexibly. Feeling supported and empowered by her own progress in her treatment already, Abigail determines that she feels prepared for clerkships and is even excited for the opportunities they will offer her to continue to combat her symptoms and striver for greater overall wellbeing.

Pearls
- Eating disorders, including AN and bulimia nervosa, as well as subclinical disordered eating, are not uncommon in the age group and population of medical students. Mental health providers working with medical students should be mindful of such disorders, comfortable with asking questions about eating and body image, and able to develop or refer to an appropriate treatment team for the student-patient with problematic eating behaviors.
- Collaboration with a team of providers, including those with expertise with using cognitive behavioral techniques and nutritional guidance for eating disorders, as well as appropriate medical support (e.g., student health services), is essential in the management of the student-patient with an eating disorder.

- The psychiatrist working with medical students with eating disorder symptoms will benefit from being aware of common stressors that can reveal or exacerbate problematic eating behaviors, as well as monitoring for countertransference experiences that can arise in working with student-patients with eating-related symptomatology.

References

1. Shisslak CM, Crago M, Estes LS. The Spectrum of eating disturbances. Int J Eat Disord. 1995;18:209–19.
2. Cotton MA, Ball C, Robinson P. Four simple questions can help screen for eating disorders. J Gen Intern Med. 2003;18:53–6.
3. Morgan JF, Reid F, Lacey H. The SCOFF questionnaire: assessment of a new screening tool for eating disorders. BMJ. 1999;319:1467–8.
4. Eisler I, Dare C, Hodes M, Russell G, Dodge E, Le Grange D. Family therapy for adolescent anorexia nervosa: the results of a controlled comparison of two family interventions. J Child Psychol Psychiatry. 2000;41:727–36.
5. Frank GK, Shott ME. The role of psychotropic medications in the management of anorexia nervosa: rationale, evidence and future prospects. CNS Drugs. 2016;30(5):419–42.

Chapter 7
The Case of Dr. Sigi Halsted: Overdose in the OR

Kristopher A. Kast and Jonathan Avery

Case

Dr. Sigi Halsted, a 34-year-old early-career anesthesiology attending, was found unconscious with shallow respirations in a staff bathroom near the operating suite where he was between surgical cases. A partially used fentanyl syringe (labeled with the name and medical record number of Dr. Halsted's recently completed case) was found nearby. After acute medical stabilization, psychiatric consultation was requested. Dr. Halsted's treatment team was concerned that this episode was a suicide attempt, but he denied this.

On initial interview Dr. Halsted—who requests to be called by his first name, Sigi—minimized the event, denying suicidal ideation, and provided a vague and inconsistent anamnesis. He reported feeling uncomfortable receiving care

K. A. Kast, MD · J. Avery, MD (✉)
Weill Cornell Medical College/New York-Presbyterian Hospital, New York, NY, USA
e-mail: kak9100@nyp.org; joa9070@med.cornell.edu

© Springer Nature Switzerland AG 2019   73
J. S. Gordon-Elliott, A. H. Rosen (eds.), *Early Career Physician Mental Health and Wellness*,
https://doi.org/10.1007/978-3-030-10952-3_7

in the hospital where he works and was preoccupied with the confidentiality of his record. His eye contact was poor, and his posture was avoidant—folded over his abdomen as if he were in pain. His affect was mildly dysphoric and irritable. He frequently sniffed or wiped his nose with clear rhinorrhea. His speech was at times interrupted by yawning. His hands were mildly tremulous bilaterally, and he was moderately hypertensive and tachycardic without clear etiology. Given his symptoms and presentation, an opioid withdrawal state was suspected, and he was largely responsive to oral buprenorphine. However, his tremulous hands and autonomic instability persisted, and alcohol withdrawal was diagnosed with persistent and tactful history gathering.

Sigi suggested that his alcohol withdrawal state was "probably" due to drinking regularly at night. He explained that he was suffering from insomnia resulting from his inconsistent shift and call schedule and alcohol helped him fall asleep. In the months leading up to this evaluation, colleagues reported intermittent absenteeism and incomplete documentation to their department leadership, though his clinical performance when present was more than adequate (and commensurate with his record of superior performance in medical school and residency) and as such nothing came of their concerns. Sigi noted that he was worried that his alcohol use was escalating but explained that he did not know how to seek help (and stated, "besides... when could I go see a doctor? I'm too busy caring for my patients"). Since residency, Sigi shared, his social network shrunk. He had few close friendships and no romantic partners. He was isolated. Additionally, he had purposefully distanced himself from his family, whom he described as an "unhealthy" group with a lot of mental health and substance use problems. He reported "sometimes" using leftover benzodiazepines or opioids from surgical cases to "rest" and manage daily anxiety or "calm my nerves" but adamantly denied using them during duty hours before his current presentation. He believed his opioid withdrawal was related to self-prescribed codeine for intermittent low-back pain, a symptom he experienced "on and off" since a minor recreational sports injury sustained during residency.

After reviewing concerns for impairment in safe medical practice, Sigi accepted a referral to the state physician health program at discharge from his emergency evaluation. He took medical leave from his practice and transferred care to a residential addiction treatment program.

Principles of Diagnosis and Management

Diagnosis

Addiction is a complex neuropsychiatric disorder with heritable risk, well-described underlying neuropathology, a relapsing disease course, characteristic effects on personality and behavior, and multiple effective treatment modalities [16]. Substance use disorders (SUD) in physicians were once considered a matter of unethical behavior subject to severe disciplinary action by licensing authorities. In 1973, the American Medical Association advocated a medical model for assessment and treatment of impaired physicians in a landmark publication [15]. The paradigm shift to conceptualizing SUD as an illness led to the development of physician health programs (PHPs) in the United States. PHPs increased access to SUD treatment for impaired physicians and allowed for physicians in recovery to return to clinical practice. PHPs now represent a standard of excellence in addiction treatment, with uniquely high rates of sustained recovery on long-term follow-up [17].

The impaired physician described in this case may be diagnosed with severe alcohol use disorder and opioid use disorder, as well as alcohol and opioid withdrawal. In DSM-5 nosology, the "substance use disorder" (SUD) syndrome includes physiologic dependence, intrapsychic preoccupation, adverse behavioral consequences, and impaired agency in changing substance use despite substance-related problems. All of these domains are present in the above case. The degree of severity is determined by the number of criteria met (see Table 7.1)[31].

TABLE 7.1 Substance use disorders: core features

Ongoing substance use in larger amounts or for a longer period of time than intended and with an inability to reduce or stop the use
Ongoing substance use despite negative implications on one's functioning (e.g., occupational, interpersonal), health, and safety
Craving for the substance, tolerance, and withdrawal

Physician impairment is not pathognomonic of SUD. Adjustment and affective disorders (unipolar and bipolar depression), among other etiologies, may lead to similar patterns of impaired professional conduct [5]. Many physicians with SUD have comorbid affective, anxiety, or personality disorders. The most common comorbidity is an affective illness plus alcohol use disorders [23]. Having both SUD and another mental disorder is associated with increased severity of impairment, persistence of both disorders, and treatment resistance [23]. Sigi, as described in the case above, has some symptoms suggestive of a comorbid anxiety or depressive disorder: insomnia, social withdrawal, lack of hedonic engagement, and subjective experience of "nerves." Further evaluation to rule out a personality disorder including antisocial personality disorder (sexual harassment, disruptive or abusive behavior, and other criminal conduct) as well as physical illness, including neurological disorders and geriatric decline, is necessary for a thorough evaluation [26]. Physical examination, screening laboratory testing, and a comprehensive forensic toxicological panel should also be performed [26]. As with all psychiatric evaluations, collateral interviews with the patient's referral source, their significant other, involved family members, and the patient's healthcare providers offer important supporting details. In the case of physician impairment, representatives of the physician's hospital or workplace environment as well as other colleagues are important collateral sources, but it is essential to handle this part of the evaluation with particular tact and attention to the patient's confidentiality.

Management and Treatment

As in Sigi's case, the impaired physician with a SUD must suspend medical practice during acute treatment [26]. This preserves the safety for the physician's patients, sustains the treatment frame for the physician-patient (which includes significant contingency management around motivation to return to clinical practice), removes access to controlled substances, and permits the intensive level of care required for standard-of-care treatment. This, concurrently, protects the impaired physician's treatment team from untoward legal risk and the potentially distressing and prohibitive countertransferential experiences of treating a patient who is placing others at risk.

The acute treatment setting for physicians newly diagnosed with SUD is usually a partial hospital or residential program with capacity for initial medical detoxification and management of withdrawal syndromes. Length of stay is typically 3 months of intensive care with individual and group psychotherapy, process groups, family therapy, recreational therapy, a psychoeducational program targeting addiction, and introduction to the 12-step program philosophy [9, 26].

The considerable out-of-pocket cost of acute intensive residential treatment can feel prohibitive for early-career physicians. The Federation of State Physician Health Programs advocates for financial planning services to assist physicians with this added challenge [2, 26].

The long-term treatment goal for physicians like Sigi in acute recovery from SUD is sustained abstinence [1, 26]. This is an ambitious outcome, and a comprehensive therapeutic frame is necessary. Participation is primarily motivated by the contingency of reporting to state licensing authorities (and potential loss of medical licensure) if the physician-patient does not comply with all the components of his or her treatment contract [26].

After acute stabilization, care is stepped down typically to biweekly outpatient care for 3–12 months and then to ongoing care management with frequent random toxicological screening, mandatory participation in community recovery support groups (e.g., Caduceus, Alcoholics/Narcotics

Anonymous, Self-Management and Recovery Training or SMART groups), and monitoring of professional functioning through workplace monitors for 5 years [20, 26].

Treatment with opioid-receptor agonists, considered the standard of care for opioid use disorders in the general population, is controversial in the physician population due to concern for potential cognitive and motor impairment. Outcomes from PHPs utilizing abstinence-based treatment show that physicians with opioid use disorder have similar outcomes to physicians with alcohol or non-opioid SUD over 5 years of intensive follow-up, suggesting that opioid-receptor agonist therapy may not be required in the physician population treated in PHPs [9]. However, for a patient with multiple opioid relapses despite compliance with intensive abstinence-based treatment, treatment may need to include opioid-receptor agonist or antagonist therapy [21,26]. Naltrexone may be preferred in physicians with opioid use disorder. However, physicians with comorbid chronic pain syndromes will often require methadone or buprenorphine treatment to manage both conditions.

Psychopharmacological management of alcohol use disorder is less controversial, and three medications are approved by the US Food and Drug Administration. Daily directly observed disulfiram dosing may be helpful for patients with engaged family or other social supports and high levels of internal motivation for abstinence. Naltrexone, dosed orally or via monthly long-acting injection, is also effective in prolonging time to relapse and reducing severity of relapses in patients with alcohol use disorder. Acamprosate may be effective in reducing craving or "anti-reward" systems mediating relief-seeking behavior via alcohol use. Additionally, topiramate and gabapentin have empirical evidence for efficacy in alcohol use disorder, though these are not FDA-approved and are associated with adverse cognitive effects [30].

Principles for Doctors Treating Doctors

SUD occur in physicians at a rate equal to the general population, with a lifetime prevalence of 8–15% and a point prevalence of 2–3.8% [1, 23, 28, 29]. Physicians most commonly present with alcohol, opioid, or benzodiazepine use disorders. Alcohol is the most common substance of abuse [1]. There is also a recent rise in cannabis use disorders with notable effects across jurisdictions with different decriminalization or legalization trends [23]. Cocaine, stimulant, hallucinogen, other sedative/hypnotic, and tobacco use disorders also occur [25].

The greatest risk factor identified among physicians with a SUD is a family history [3]. There is also evidence for some risk associated with higher academic performance and narcissistic or obsessive-compulsive personality traits [1, 3, 13]. Excessive alcohol use among medical students had no impact on clinical rotation performance consistent with the hypothesis that deterioration in the workplace is a late finding among physicians with SUD [1]. This likely contributes to a known delay in SUD identification and treatment [2, 23, 24]. Typically, alcohol abuse presents earliest with high rates of alcohol abuse/dependence in medical student populations. Risk of problematic alcohol use in medical school is even higher in cases with comorbid depression, professional burnout, single marital status, younger age, and high educational debt [11]. Abuse of opioids and sedative/hypnotics among young physicians typically begins during residency training once physicians have prescribing privileges. In these situations, physicians classically report initiating usage by self-prescribing for "treatment" rather than for recreation [7]. Rates of mood and anxiety disorders are greater in physicians than the general population. Physicians are often struggling with untreated mental illness and concurrently less likely to be in the care of other physicians (for both medical and psychiatric illnesses). This contributes to prevalent self-prescribing [20].

Some medical specialties, specifically emergency medicine and anesthesiology, are overrepresented in SUD treatment. Emergency medicine has a nearly threefold higher rate of admission to treatment programs [4]. Anesthesiology is also overrepresented and associated with more frequent opioid use and intravenous route of use of substances [10, 12].

Mortality is markedly elevated among physicians with SUD [6, 8, 12]. These deaths are due to overdose, medical complications of the SUD, and suicide. Completed physician suicides have been associated with alcohol intoxication, SUD diagnosis, and self-prescription of medication by the suicide completer [1]. Additional, though not fatal, risks associated with physician SUD include legal repercussions (e.g., driving while intoxicated) and increased interpersonal conflict with family and colleagues [21].

It must be emphasized that SUD diagnosis and functional impairment are distinct but related issues [18, 19]. Untreated SUD typically progresses to physician impairment, but early identification and intervention may lead to recovery before impairment occurs. The window of opportunity between illness onset and impairment may be greater than 6 years in the physician population [2, 23, 24], but potent barriers limit early referral. These include prevalent denial-based unconscious defenses, stigma-motivated conscious concealment, aversion to assuming the patient role, concerns related to obtaining practice cross coverage during treatment (or reluctance to remove oneself from medical practice or "abandon patients"), and fear of disciplinary action from licensing boards [19].

A consequence of a punitive approach to physician impairment, once the standard practice among state licensing boards, led to frequent delay to identification of illness and treatment. Ill physicians were wary to risk the far-reaching consequences of permanently suspended medical licensure, and concerned colleagues similarly balked at these high stakes when considering intervention [27]. The legacy of a criminal or moral failing model of understanding substance use rather than a medical model is hypothesized to lead to more physicians with SUD avoiding treatment, exposing patients to potential risk, and physicians progressing to functional impairment [19]. In Sigi's case, colleagues noted troubling behavior before his overdose at work. This was a missed opportunity for early intervention.

The American Medical Association and the Federation of State Medical Boards advocate for ill physicians to receive voluntary, confidential treatment while maintaining adequate safeguards to protect public safety. Physician health programs (PHPs) are independent third parties organized by the state medical boards or medical societies to manage evaluation, referral to treatment, and subsequent monitoring. PHPs provide posttreatment relapse monitoring for up to 5 years to ensure stability of recovery with return to clinical practice [20, 26]. Several other nations have modeled their systems after these effective programs [20].

Physician-patients are either self-referred or referred by colleagues or administrators to PHPs. Self-referred physicians are usually able to participate confidentially, without involvement of state licensing authorities. Impaired physicians who decline to participate in the PHP-monitored evaluation and treatment or who are unable to maintain adequate stability of recovery are subject to legal repercussions and loss of medical licensure.

Initial clinical presentations of physicians with SUD vary widely. The most commonly reported presentations include self-identification of risky use or early use disorder, nonspecific abnormal workplace behavior, poor or incomplete documentation, absenteeism, witnessed substance use or intoxication in the workplace (varying from odor of alcohol on the breath to observed intravenous injection of hospital opioids), and death by accidental or intentional overdose [12]. Notably, some physicians with SUD will demonstrate more behavioral signs of impairment when the substance is absent (i.e., in a state of withdrawal or craving and preoccupation) than when it is present [29].

It is an ethical obligation, and in most jurisdictions a legal requirement, to report impaired physician-colleagues to appropriate state medical boards or to the state's PHP [14, 22]. This protects public health and safety while ensuring the ill physician receives appropriate evaluation and treatment for a potentially lethal disorder.

Identifying concerning behavior in a colleague (or oneself) precedes and is separate from the assessment of a physician-patient within the context of a forensic or therapeutic relationship; it is ill-advised to serve both roles. Concerned colleagues or administrators should first gather and record factual observations that are cause for concern. These are required for the first step in an "intervention" for a potentially ill colleague. The FRAMER acronym highlights intervention steps ([2, 29]; see Table 7.2). Ideally, an intervention should be launched in concert with their state PHP [26].

The goal of this kind of intervention is mutual agreement to immediate cessation of medical practice, evaluation and treatment of the physician-patient, and duly documented impairment in functioning. Referral to the state PHP or medical board must occur in accordance with jurisdictional statutes, regardless of the impaired physician's decision to comply.

TABLE 7.2 Framing an intervention for an impaired colleague: the FRAMER acronym mnemonic

Facts: Gather and document the factual observations of the physician's behavior leading to concern for impairment

Responsibility: Determine the mandated legal responsibility for reporting suspected impairment; this varies by state jurisdiction

Another person: Bring a representative of the state PHP to the meeting with the impaired physician; this person may serve as a witness to the conversation and serve as a resource for information regarding next steps

Monologue: Begin the intervention with a complete, matter-of-fact list of the observations leading to concern (gathered during the "Facts" step above); the meeting is an intervention, not a debate

Evaluation: A comprehensive, independent evaluation must occur, and the physician should immediately cease practice during the evaluation and treatment (meaning cross-coverage should be arranged for the physician's patients)

Report back: Ensure pertinent findings and recommended treatment from the evaluation are able to be provided to the concerned parties, including those administratively involved in the physician's practice

Adapted from Boyd [2]

Outcomes

Positive outcomes, including sustained remission and return to clinical practice, occur in 70–80% of physicians treated by PHPs over a 5-year follow-up [1, 4, 8]. This is an extraordinarily high success rate and a cause for optimism in treating physicians with SUD. Outcomes in populations without access to PHPs are less positive. In an Australian-New Zealander population of anesthesiologists, only 32% of identified physician-patients successfully returned to work following largely outpatient-based short-duration treatment for SUD [12]. Rates of response to intensive SUD treatment within PHPs do not differ between physician-patients of different medical specialties [4, 10].

Prevention is of paramount importance. Recommendations to prevent development of SUD are based largely on an epidemiological understanding of risk factors and good sense. Self-prescription of medication by physicians should be indiscriminately avoided. Ensuring physicians are able to tend to personal medical and psychological health is critical. This may curtail self-treatment, as well. Regular healthcare appointments, adequate exercise, participation in self-directed leisure activities, and engagement in nonmedical social activities should all be promoted by training programs and departmental leadership [2].

Pearls
- Impairment is not equivalent to a diagnosis of SUD.
- Impairment in the workplace is usually a late finding in physicians with SUD; a colleague's worrisome behavior in the healthcare environment should trigger concern for escalating (rather than early) functional impairment.
- Physicians with SUD have an elevated risk of all-cause mortality; completed physician suicides are often associated with SUD, alcohol intoxication, and self-prescription of medication by the suicide completer.

- Treatment of physicians with SUD occurs through the supervision and case management of state PHPs, which act as diversion programs to avoid loss of medical licensure.
- Outcomes are remarkably positive for physicians with SUD treated through state PHPs, with a majority of physicians experiencing sustained recovery and return to clinical practice over an extended follow-up.

References

1. Earley PH. Physician health programs and addiction among physicians. In: Ries RK, Fiellin DA, Miller SC, Saitz R, editors. The ASAM principles of addiction medicine. 5th ed. New York: Wolters Kluwer; 2014.
2. Boyd JW, Knight JR. Substance use disorders among physicians. In: Galanter M, Kleber HD, Brady KT, editors. The American Psychiatric Publishing Textbook of substance abuse treatment, 5th Edition. American Psychiatric Publishing. 2015. https://psychiatryonline.org/doi/full/10.1176/appi.books.9781615370030.mg46. Accessed 1 Nov 2017.
3. Flaherty JA, Richman JA. Substance use and addiction among medical students, residents, and physicians. Psychiatr Clin North Am. 1993;16(1):189–97.
4. Rose JS, Campbell M, Skipper G. Prognosis for emergency physician with substance abuse recovery: 5-year outcome study. West J Emerg Med. 2014;15(1):20–5.
5. Brown SD, Goske MJ, Johnson CM. Beyond substance abuse: stress, burnout, and depression as causes of physician impairment and disruptive behavior. J Am Coll Radiol. 2009;6(7):479–85.
6. Yarborough WH. Substance use disorders in physician training programs. J Okla State Med Assoc. 1999;92(10):504–7.
7. Hughes PH, Conard SE, Baldwin DC Jr, Storr CL, Sheehan DV. Resident physician substance use in the United States. JAMA. 1991;265(16):2069–73.

8. McLellan AT, Skipper GS, Campbell M, DuPont RL. Five year outcomes in a cohort study of physicians treated for substance use disorders in the United States. BMJ. 2008;337:a2038.
9. Merlo LJ, Campbell MD, Skipper GE, Shea CL, DuPont RL. Outcomes for physicians with opioid dependence treated without agonist pharmacotherapy in physician health programs. J Subst Abus Treat. 2016;64:47–54.
10. Skipper GE, Campbell MD, Dupont RL. Anesthesiologists with substance use disorders: a 5-year outcome study from 16 state physician health programs. Anesth Analg. 2009;109(3):891–6.
11. Jackson ER, Shanafelt TD, Hasan O, Satele DV, Dyrbye LN. Burnout and alcohol abuse/dependence among U.S. medical students. Acad Med. 2016;91(9):1251–6.
12. Fry RA, Fry LE, Castanelli DJ. A retrospective survey of substance abuse in anesthetists in Australia and New Zealand from 2004 to 2013. Anaesth Intensive Care. 2015;43(1):111–7.
13. Clark DC, Daugherty SR. A norm-referenced longitudinal study of medical student drinking patterns. J Subst Abuse. 1990;2:15–37.
14. Sudan R, Seymour K. The impaired surgeon. Surg Clin N Am. 2016;96:89–93.
15. The sick physician: impairment by psychiatric disorders, including alcoholism and drug dependence. JAMA. 1973;223(6):684–7.
16. Koob GF. Neurobiology of addiction. In: Galanter M, Kleber HD, Brady KT, editors. Textbook of substance abuse treatment, 5th Edition. American Psychiatric Publishing; 2015. https://psychiatryonline.org/doi/full/10.1176/appi.books.9781615370030.mg01. Accessed 15 Oct 2017.
17. DuPont RL, McLellan AT, White WL, et al. Setting the standard for recovery: physicians' health programs. J Subst Abus Treat. 2009;36(2):159–71.
18. Policy on physician impairment. Federation of State Medical Boards. 2011. https://www.fsmb.org/Media/Default/PDF/FSMB/Advocacy/grpol_policy-on-physician-impairment.pdf. Accessed 1 Nov 2017.
19. Public policy statement: physician illness vs. impairment. Federation of State Physician Health Programs. 2008. https://www.fsmb.org/Media/Default/PDF/FSMB/Advocacy/grpol_policy-on-physician-impairment.pdf. Accessed 1 Nov 2017.
20. Braquehais MD, Tresidder A, DuPont RL. Service provision to physicians with mental health and addiction problems. Curr Opin Psychiatry. 2015;28:324–9.

21. Merlo LJ, Gold MS. Prescription opioid abuse and dependence among physicians: hypotheses and treatment. Harv Rev Psychiatry. 2008;16:181–94.
22. Physician responsibilities to impaired colleagues. In: Code of Medical Ethics Opinion 9.3.2. American Medical Association. 2016. https://www.ama-assn.org/delivering-care/physician-responsibilities-impaired-colleagues. Accessed 1 Nov 2017.
23. Braquehais MD, Lusilla P, Bel MJ, Navarro MC, Nasillo V, Diaz A, Valero S, Padros J, Bruguera E, Casas M. Dual diagnosis among physicians: a clinical perspective. J Dual Diagn. 2014;10(3):148–55.
24. Brooke D, Edwards G, Taylor C. Addiction as an occupational hazard: 144 doctors with drug and alcohol problems. Addiction. 1991;86(8):1011–6.
25. Galanter M, Dermatis H, Mansch P, McIntyre J, Perez-Fuentes G. Substance-abusing physicians: monitoring and twelve-step-based treatment. Am J Addict. 2007;16:117–23.
26. Physician health program guidelines. Federation of State Physician Health Programs. 2005. http://www.fsphp.org/sites/default/files/pdfs/2005_fsphp_guidelines-master_0.pdf. Accessed 30 Oct 2017.
27. Weiss Roberts L, Warner TD, Rogers M, Horwitz R, Redgrave G. Medical student illness and impairment: a vignette-based survey study involved 955 students at 9 medical schools. Compr Psychiatry. 2005;46:229–37.
28. Oreskovich MR, Shanafelt T, Dyrbye LN, Tan L, Sotile W, Satele D, West CP, Sloan J, Boone S. The prevalence of substance use disorders in American physicians. Am J Addict. 2015;24:30–8.
29. Knight JR. A 35-year-old physician with opioid dependence. JAMA. 2004;292(11):1351–7.
30. Reus VI, Fochtmann LJ, Bukstein O, Eyler AE, Hilty DM, Horvitz-Lennon M, Mahoney J, Pasic J, Weaver M, Wills CD, McIntyre J, Kidd J, Yager J, Hong S-H. The American Psychiatric Association practice guideline for the pharmacological treatment of patients with alcohol use disorder. Am J Psychiatry. 2018;175:86–90.
31. Substance-related and addictive disorders. In: Diagnostic and statistical manual of mental disorders, Fifth Edition. American Psychiatric Publishing; 2013. https://dsm.psychiatryonline.org/doi/full/10.1176/appi.books.9780890425596.dsm16. Accessed 15 Oct 2017.

Chapter 8
The Case of Erik Quimby: A Disruptive Physician in Training

Daniel Knoepflmacher

Case

Erik Quimby, a 28-year-old, third-year resident in a competitive surgical specialty at a well-known academic hospital, was evaluated by Dr. Davis, an attending psychiatrist who regularly treats residents. Erik's program director referred him after a series of complaints were lodged against him by fellow residents, attendings, and medical staff.

Upon first seeing Dr. Davis, Erik explained that their meeting was "a big mistake" because he had been "unfairly targeted." He denied any prior psychiatric treatment but claimed to know a lot about psychiatry, having earned the highest grade in his third-year clerkship at a top-rated medical school. He methodically ruled out various psychiatric diagnoses, delineating how none of the criteria for several "Axis I" disorders applied to him. He described working out regularly, drinking rarely, and abstaining from substance use in order to "maintain my top form." Dr. Davis, who said little during the first 15 minutes of their encounter, asked Erik to explain why his program director had referred him.

D. Knoepflmacher, MD, MFA (✉)
Weill Cornell Medical College/New York-Presbyterian Hospital,
New York, NY, USA
e-mail: dak9065@med.cornell.edu

© Springer Nature Switzerland AG 2019   87
J. S. Gordon-Elliott, A. H. Rosen (eds.), *Early Career Physician Mental Health and Wellness*,
https://doi.org/10.1007/978-3-030-10952-3_8

Erik became visibly frustrated as he described a "conspiracy" against him. His narrative became more disjointed, punctuated by several angry accusations. He claimed a senior resident on his last rotation was "threatened" by him. He believed she became jealous after an esteemed attending surgeon on their team repeatedly complimented Erik's surgical technique and depth of knowledge. He claimed she then "ganged up" on him with a surgical technician and a nurse, both of whom had also complained about him. When asked how he treated the technician and the nurse, he admitted raising his voice occasionally when they failed to follow his directions. He felt this was appropriate, pointing to "the hierarchy," where all subordinate staff should "respect" his status as a surgeon and "make sure to do their job the right way."

Dr. Davis asked if there might be other reasons why the senior resident and the staff reacted negatively towards him. After a moment he responded, "I can be direct, but they were out to get me." Dr. Davis disclosed that Erik's program director had reported a longstanding history of behavior problems, with frequent angry outbursts. He listed several episodes that had been reported to him by the program director, including "a pattern" of openly defying certain surgical attendings, being aggressive with consulting physicians from other specialties, arguing loudly with peers in front of patients, and a recent episode where he threw a soiled linen at a janitor who he said was being "too loud." Responding to this, Erik became visibly angry. In an expletive-laden tirade, he complained about being victimized. He accused Dr. Davis of being "some shrink who just doesn't get it." He eventually revealed that he was being forced to take a mandatory leave of absence, which was "humiliating." Unable to hold back tears, he said he wasn't sure what he would do if he were kicked out of the residency. Dr. Davis asked him about suicidal or homicidal thoughts. Erik denied current ideation, but added that if his career as a surgeon were taken away from him, his life would "have no purpose."

Dr. Davis expressed an empathic response to Erik's predicament, reflecting how Erik's lifelong dream must have felt as if it were in jeopardy. Erik agreed with this, gradually regaining his composure. He completed the rest of the evaluation, agreed to submit samples for blood and urine tests, and promised to follow up with Dr. Davis. As he got up from his chair at the end of the session, he made close eye contact with Dr. Davis, "I'm a surgeon. It's what I was always meant to be." Reaching over to pat Dr. Davis on the shoulder, he added, "We'll show them I'm not crazy," and walked out the door.

Principles of Diagnosis and Management

Diagnosis

In their 2009 book, *The Physician as Patient: A Clinical Handbook for Mental Health Professionals*, Myers and Gabbard suggest that the term "disruptive physician" is often a euphemism used to describe a doctor with a personality disorder [1]. Despite a wide differential diagnosis in the case of Erik, one can clearly identify several facets of the DSM-5 diagnostic criteria for narcissistic personality disorder [2]; see Table 8.1. Other Cluster B personality disorder diagnoses, such as borderline or antisocial personality disorder, should

TABLE 8.1 Features of narcissistic personality disorder commonly found in disruptive physician behavior

"exhibits a pattern of grandiosity (in fantasy or behavior), need for admiration, and lack of empathy."

"expects to be recognized as superior without commensurate achievements"

"is preoccupied with fantasies of unlimited success"

"believes he is 'special'...should only associate with other special or high-status people"

"has a sense of entitlement."

"believes that others are envious of him"

"shows arrogant, haughty behaviors or attitudes."

be considered when evaluating physicians with aggressive behavior problems. On further questioning during a follow-up session, Dr. Davis did not detect adequate evidence for either of these diagnoses. Specifically, Erik did not describe or manifest behavior consistent with unstable identity, fear of abandonment, feelings of emptiness, impulsivity, chronic suicidality, or self-injurious behaviors that are common in borderline personality disorder, nor did his history fully match the pattern of irresponsibility, unethical behavior, impulsivity, reckless disregard for safety, or deceitfulness characteristic of antisocial personality disorder. Erik exhibits some of the perfectionism and rigidity commonly seen in obsessive-compulsive personality disorder. While these traits would be important to keep in mind during treatment, they do not fully explain the pathological behaviors behind his presenting problems.

Outside of the personality disorder realm, intermittent explosive disorder (IED) is another DSM-5 diagnosis that describes Erik's difficulties controlling his anger. The diagnostic criteria include "recurrent behavioral outbursts representing a failure to control aggressive impulses," "verbal aggression (e.g., temper tantrums, tirades, verbal arguments or fights) or physical aggression" occurring "twice weekly, on average, for a period of 3 months." Erik meets these criteria and the general standard of "impairment in occupational or interpersonal functioning," given that the behavior has begun to cause problems for him in, at least, his professional life. As described in the DSM-5, IED can follow a more episodic, recurrent pattern, which could explain how someone like Erik might perform better in certain environments at certain times (e.g., medical school) but run into more behavioral impairment in other contexts with a different range of stressors and role functions (e.g., surgery residency).

The combined diagnoses of narcissistic personality disorder and intermittent explosive disorder are especially disabling in his case, creating a serious threat to his deeply held career goals, not to mention the safety of his patients and co-workers. Individuals with IED might feel remorse or distress after an explosive episode, but someone with Erik's underlying character pathology feels justified instead. Lacking the necessary insight for corrective self-evaluation, he has a reflexive tendency to project blame on to others and little to no ability to empathize with the internal experiences of those he attacks.

In rounding out the differential diagnosis, primary disorders of mood, especially bipolar disorder, should be considered as a possible cause of Erik's reported symptoms. On Dr. Davis' assessment, this seemed unlikely. He lacks a clear history of mania, hypomania, or depressive episodes. Though he does not meet the criteria for major depression, his tearful and anxious reaction to the threat of being thrown out of his residency could be early evidence of an adjustment disorder, something that could be assessed further in follow-up sessions.

Erik denied significant alcohol and substance use. Patients often fail to fully disclose their substance use during medical or psychiatric evaluations. For someone like Erik, undergoing a high-stakes evaluation with major implications for his career, there is an even greater incentive to conceal. Certainly, stimulant or cocaine use should always be considered when evaluating disruptive or erratic behavior in physicians. One would look out for positive results on random urine screens or corroborating signs on successive mental status exams. Anabolic steroid use, or other performance-enhancing substances that might be used by an individual looking to build muscle, may similarly contribute to impulsive and aggressive behavior and should be considered and screened for, especially in light of Erik's reported interest in "working out" and optimizing his physique.

Dr. Davis obtained consent from Erik for a urine toxicology screen and blood tests. Laboratory results, along with a detailed medical history and basic physical exam, can help rule out other possible but less likely factors (e.g., hyperthyroidism, traumatic brain injury, seizure history, medication side effects).

Management and Treatment

Narcissistic personality disorder is a notoriously difficult diagnosis to treat, requiring long-term psychotherapy (e.g., mentalization-based treatment, transference-focused psychotherapy, schema-focused psychotherapy, or psychodynamic psychotherapy) by skilled clinicians. The case of Erik, however, requires a more acute intervention. While it's helpful to be mindful of the underlying personality pathology, the initial phase of treatment must be focused on managing the behavioral problems that are threatening his ability to continue his training and potentially putting patients and others at risk. In this case, the secondary diagnosis of IED provides evidence for acute and time-limited treatment.

Clinical research on IED is limited, but there is evidence for both psychotherapeutic and pharmacological treatments in individuals struggling with anger management problems. Whether or not medications are indicated as part of the treatment, a course of goal-oriented psychotherapy can provide a framework for overall management. There is evidence, both from several meta-analytic studies and one clinical trial, that cognitive behavioral therapy (CBT) with a focus on managing anger is an effective modality for reducing impulsive aggression [3]. CBT treatment in this context may include relaxation training, cognitive restructuring, and an integration of adaptive coping skills. Dialectical behavioral therapy (DBT), with its efficacy in reducing both impulsivity and anger, is another appropriate psychotherapeutic modality [4].

As the case of Erik illustrates, impulsive and aggressive patients present a risk for suicidal and homicidal ideation. Erik conveys uncertainty about how he might react to the narcissistic injury he fears most, being terminated from his residency. In a case such as this one, the risks of suicide and workplace violence should be continuously evaluated during treatment, along with therapeutic interventions to help the patient appropriately cope with distress. If the risk of any potentially harmful behavior is identified, a safety plan outlining concrete steps to reduce risk should be established in collaboration with the patient [5].

With a framework for psychotherapy established, various pharmacological interventions can be used to help regulate the emotional and behavioral symptoms of IED. The neuropathophysiology of impulsive aggression has been linked to reductions of serotonin in the prefrontal cortex, making serotonin reuptake inhibitors (SRIs) logical candidates for clinical trials. The efficacy of fluoxetine was investigated in two double-blind, placebo-controlled studies, one specifically targeting patients with intermittent explosive disorder and another focused on treating aggressive behavior in personality-disordered individuals [6, 7]. Results in both showed a significant reduction in measurable aggression when subjects were treated with fluoxetine. Other SRIs, which have been studied in this context even less thoroughly than fluoxetine, are generally accepted as equivalent choices for treating IED. SRIs should be particularly favored when the aggressive symptoms co-occur with depression, anxiety, or compulsive behavior.

Antiseizure medications (e.g., divalproex, carbamazepine, oxcarbazepine, phenytoin) have also been used to treat impulsive aggression [8], but many of these come with significant side effects, some of which could impair work that demands operational precision, such as surgery. Lamotrigine is a reasonable option in this case, with its relatively low side effect profile and evidence of efficacy for treating impulsive aggression in borderline personality disorder patients [9]. With any significant suspicion of bipolar spectrum symptoms, it may be preferable to start with a mood stabilizer instead of an SRI. Other pharmacological options that have shown some evidence of efficacy in treating intermittent explosive disorder include beta-blockers (propranolol), alpha-2 agonists (clonidine and guanfacine), and atypical antipsychotics (aripiprazole, quetiapine) [10], though several of these medications could also cause potentially impairing side effects.

Principles for Doctors Treating Doctors

Although not a formal diagnosis, the term "disruptive physician" has become a common way to describe doctors behaving badly in the medical setting. In 2009, the Joint Commission issued a Sentinel Event Alert statement entitled "Behaviors that undermine a culture of safety." In this document, they highlight the widespread prevalence and significant associated risk of disruptive behavior in healthcare. To address this problem, they provide a series of requirements and suggested actions, which include adopting a "zero tolerance" for "intimidating and disruptive behaviors" into medical staff bylaws [11]. With these increased efforts to maintain professionalism, many physicians may be compelled into seeking mental health treatment they might otherwise avoid.

The Accreditation Council for Graduate Medical Education (ACGME) mandates that professionalism and interpersonal communication skills be included as core competencies for residency training [12]. If training leadership identifies a resident exhibiting disruptive behavior, it must first be assessed whether the behavior is potentially amenable to remediation, and a plan to do so should be developed. Without improvement, residents may not be promoted or, in rarer cases, are forced to leave the training program. A clinician, such as Dr. Davis, needs to be aware of the role of the mental health provider in an organization's administrative policies for addressing disruptive physicians (see Fig. 8.1).

The overarching administrative process provides parameters for remediation, some of which can complement the treatment provided by the clinician caring for a disruptive physician. Often, physicians in treatment for aggressive behavior are mandated to attend a comprehensive program that provides intensive behavioral education and adaptive coping strategies [13]. Several of these programs exist around the country, including those at Vanderbilt University, the University of Virginia, and the University of California. While these programs can be beneficial elements of the treatment and remediation process, they are typically short-term inter-

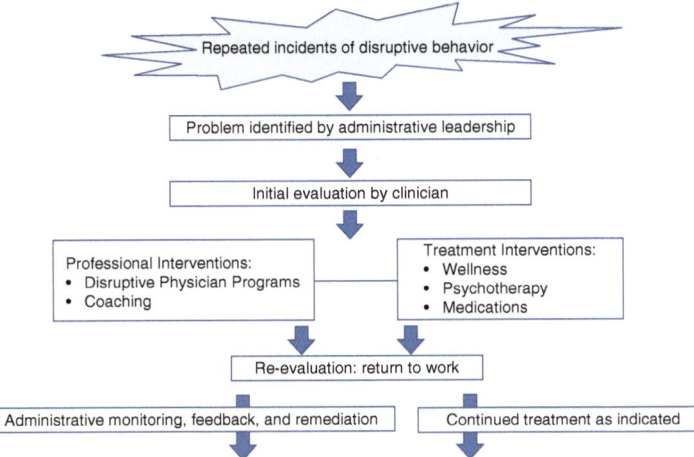

Figure 8.1 Organizational pathway for the identification, treatment, and remediation of disruptive physicians

ventions that need continual reinforcement once the individual returns to the workplace. Successfully supporting the long-term behavioral stability of physicians in treatment requires ongoing coordination of therapeutic and professional support within their local environment.

The psychiatrist treating the disruptive physician is confronted with the inherent tension between therapeutic and administrative demands. The role of the provider often has several overlapping domains: treating the physician-patient while determining whether they are fit to return to duty, maintaining confidentiality while needing to maintain contact with administrative leadership, and working to ensure the physician-patient's safety while also attending to the safety of the physician's patients and colleagues (see Fig. 8.2). While these goals may align, they often present conflicts between competing ethical principles (e.g., autonomy vs. beneficence, duty to the individual vs. the community). In some cases, these inherent conflicts can be eliminated by assigning the potentially conflicting roles to different individuals. One provider can complete the forensic evaluation

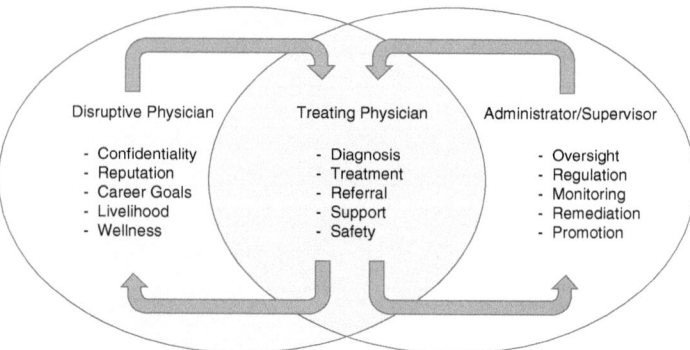

FIGURE 8.2 Overlapping demands in the treatment of disruptive physicians

determining fitness for duty, while another only provides treatment. This can allow a fitness evaluator to avoid additional bias that may come from a drive to create therapeutic rapport with the patient. The treatment provider, on the other hand, must always remain aware of potential administrative concerns. In the case of Erik, Dr. Davis did not have the luxury of having another psychiatrist to fulfill the purely forensic role. Erik points to this tension when he suggests, somewhat aggressively, that Dr. Davis will need to let his program director know he is "not crazy," alluding to the fact that Dr. Davis is responsible for determining whether Erik will be fit to return to work as a resident while simultaneously trying to maintain a therapeutic alliance.

Often medical students or residents come in for an evaluation with background information provided to the psychiatrist by administrative leadership beforehand, which can impede the physician-patient's full cooperation and disclosure. As in the case of Erik, the physician patient may only be seeing a psychiatrist because administrative leadership compelled them to be evaluated. Special care must be taken to introduce collateral information in a way that can elicit the full story from the patient without unduly increasing any underlying paranoia or distrust. Whenever possible, it is helpful to maintain openness about necessary communication to and from outside administrators throughout the course of treatment. Dr. Davis disclosed the background information provided by Erik's program director after initially letting Erik describe why he thought he was sent in. In setting the frame for continuing treatment, Dr. Davis could build on this initial disclosure by describing how he would inform Erik about future communications with the program director, highlighting how the vast majority of material from ongoing treatment would remain confidential. When treating disruptive physicians, setting clear boundaries for confidentiality and disclosure avoids blindsiding the patient, helps to build trust, and is fundamental for creating and preserving a therapeutic alliance.

When confronting the complex dynamics of treating a disruptive physician, it is helpful to maintain awareness of the transference and countertransference reactions that will naturally arise. Erik vacillates between demeaning Dr. Davis as "some shrink" to accepting his empathy as someone who understands what he's going through. Given that the treatment of disruptive physicians often involves the combination of a high-stakes context with underlying personality pathology in the patient, one can expect a wide range of intense transferences on the part of the physician-patient, ranging from aggressive minimization to adoring idealization. The treating psychiatrist must attend to their own countertransference, being mindful of ways in which they might overidentify with a fellow physician in crisis or generate aggressive reactions to the patient's narcissism. As with all challenging cases, supervision from a skilled colleague can be helpful in managing complicated countertransference and even potentially utilizing the information gleaned from countertransference responses to enhance the delivery of treatment.

Outcome

During his medical leave, Erik completed a comprehensive treatment program for disruptive physicians and engaged in weekly treatment. Dr. Davis started fluoxetine and provided supportive psychotherapy. Erik forged a therapeutic alliance with Dr. Davis, which helped him understand how his interpersonal conflicts and aggressive emotional responses were jeopardizing his career goals.

Upon returning to work, he was monitored as part of a remediation plan designed by his program director. He was required to meet with supervisors for regular feedback sessions, where he was evaluated on his performance and professionalism. Despite the extra scrutiny, he had no recurrence of aggressive outbursts.

He continued to see Dr. Davis intermittently over the next 6 months, successfully meeting the requirements of the remediation plan. That July, when Erik entered into a research year, Dr. Davis referred him to a psychologist specializing in mentalization-based treatment. Though initially reluctant to see someone new, Erik had developed more curiosity about himself over the preceding months of treatment and remediation and agreed to try. He learned to value this different approach to therapy as he gained an understanding of how other people experienced his aggressive emotional reactions. He continued psychotherapy and medications through the remainder of residency, after which he successfully matched into a competitive surgical oncology fellowship.

Pearls
- Consider cluster B personality disorders, bipolar disorder, intermittent explosive disorder, and substance use disorders when evaluating disruptive physicians.
- When treating disruptive physicians with personality disorder diagnoses, address treatable symptoms and modifiable disruptive behaviors as the primary focus for acute treatment. Long-term therapy may be indicated to address underlying character pathology.
- Serotonin reuptake inhibitors and mood stabilizers are mainstays of pharmacological treatment for impulsive aggression and intermittent explosive dis-

order, but physicians must be mindful of side effects that could impair the physician-patient's performance at work.

- CBT and DBT are useful therapeutic modalities in the treatment of disruptive physicians with emotional regulation problems or IED.
- Psychiatrists treating disruptive physicians must carefully manage the potential conflicts that can arise between administrative responsibilities and therapeutic goals. Clear boundaries and a framework for disclosure and confidentiality should be established early and reinforced continually throughout treatment.

References

1. Myers MF, Gabbard GO. The physician as patient: a clinical handbook for mental health professionals. Washington, DC: American Psychiatric Pub; 2009.
2. American Psychiatric Association. Diagnostic and statistical manual of mental disorders. 5th ed. Arlington: American Psychiatric Publishing; 2013.
3. McCloskey MS, Noblett KL, Deffenbacher JL, Gollan JK, Coccaro EF. Cognitive-behavioral therapy for intermittent explosive disorder: a pilot randomized clinical trial. J Consult Clin Psychol. 2008;76(5):876.
4. Hollander E, Stein DJ, editors. Clinical manual of impulse-control disorders. Washington, DC: American Psychiatric Pub; 2007.
5. Stanley B, Brown GK. Safety planning intervention: a brief intervention to mitigate suicide risk. Cogn Behav Pract. 2012;19(2):256–64.
6. Coccaro EF, Kavoussi RJ. Fluoxetine and impulsive aggressive behavior in personality-disordered subjects. Arch Gen Psychiatry. 1997;54:1081–8.
7. Coccaro EF, Lee RJ, Kavoussi RJ. A double-blind, randomized, placebo-controlled trial of fluoxetine in patients with intermittent explosive disorder. J Clin Psychiatry. 2009;70:653–62.

8. Stanford MS, Anderson NE, Lake SL, Baldridge RM. Pharmacologic treatment of impulsive aggression with anti-epileptic drugs. Curr Treat Options Neurol. 2009;11(5):383–90.

9. Tritt K, Nickel C, Lahmann C, Leiberich PK, Rother WK, Loew TH, Nickel MK. Lamotrigine treatment of aggression in female borderline-patients: a randomized, double-blind, placebo-controlled study. J Psychopharmacol. 2005;19(3):287–91.

10. Olvera RL. Intermittent explosive disorder. CNS Drugs. 2002;16(8):517–26.

11. Alert SE. Behaviors that undermine a culture of safety. Sentinel Event Alert. 2008(40):1–3.

12. Accreditation Council for Graduate Medical Education. ACGME common program requirements. 2013.

13. Swiggart WH, Dewey CM, Hickson GB, Finlayson AR, Spickard WA Jr. A plan for identification, treatment, and remediation of disruptive behaviors in physicians. Front Health Serv Manag. 2009;25(4):3.

Suggested Reading

Vukmir RB. Disruptive healthcare provider behavior: an evidence-based guide. Cham: Springer; 2016.

Chapter 9
The Case of Tammy Dohada: When a Fellow Resident and Close Friend Commits Suicide

Anna Miari

Case

Dr. Tammy Dohada was 29 years old and at the start of her second year of residency in pediatrics in a large tertiary care medical center when she consulted Dr. Singer, a House Staff Mental Health Program psychiatrist, within the same hospital.

Upon entering Dr. Singer's office, Tammy quickly scanned the room and Dr. Singer's facial expression and then slowly sat down. She made good eye contact but appeared slightly guarded. In a soft voice and with little emotion on her face she said, "My attending told me I should talk to someone." Upon further inquiry, she explained, "I have not been doing well since my friend died. She killed herself. A friend of mine is also upset, she had thoughts of suicide, and came to see someone in the program here…I am not sure this will help me."

A. Miari, MD (✉)
Weill Cornell Medical College/New York-Presbyterian Hospital, New York, NY, USA
e-mail: anm2004@med.cornell.edu

© Springer Nature Switzerland AG 2019   101
J. S. Gordon-Elliott, A. H. Rosen (eds.), *Early Career Physician Mental Health and Wellness*,
https://doi.org/10.1007/978-3-030-10952-3_9

Since her friend Rebecca's suicide, about 6 weeks prior, Tammy reported experiencing intense anger, sadness, and anxiety. She described feeling newly mistrustful of her superiors. She frequently questioned their clinical judgment and challenged it directly, at times with an arrogant tone. She was anxious, compulsively looked up literature about her cases, and stayed late at work double-checking her own orders and writing meticulous notes. Tammy believed that her work performance was not the same, though no one had expressed any specific concerns. Despite tiredness, she had difficulty falling asleep and getting out of bed in the morning. She had arrived late a few mornings to rounds, but, to her surprise, she had not cared – "it's not like anyone notices." Her concentration at work was diminished. She was alarmed about having once forgotten to write an order for an antibiotic for one of her inpatients. Fortunately the resident on call caught the mistake and no harm occurred. She was often distracted by angry blaming thoughts, alternatively blaming the hospital for having failed her friend, or blaming herself for not having been able to prevent the suicide. Her friend Rebecca had developed depression during their internship together; Tammy had encouraged her to seek psychiatric help, which she did, and recently she seemed to be improving. "I cannot believe she didn't say anything to me before she did this…Her doctor works here. You cannot trust anyone…I thought this could not happen at this hospital. This is supposed to be a good hospital. We are supposed to take care of other people, but nobody is taking care of us. I don't know if I can continue to work here." She asked whether Dr. Singer knew the psychiatrist who had been treating her friend.

Tammy had been wondering about taking a leave of absence, and even thought of quitting medicine entirely. In this context, she revealed that when she was 11 years old, while attending sleepaway camp for the first time, her middle brother died at age 8 of septicemia while hospitalized. She had been aware that this traumatic life event both inspired and generated ambivalence about her choice to become a physician. She denied any personal history of a psychiatric disorder or problematic substance use, though she offhandedly described to Dr. Singer a period during college "when I was just being superficial, and I wasn't really eating and I was exercising too much; oh, it wasn't a big deal – my friends said they wanted to help, but I got it under control, myself." A high-achieving student and with a major in education, Tammy took time off after college and worked for Teach for America while resolving her doubts before enrolling in medical school.

As Dr. Singer was listening, memories of an instance of suicide by a fellow resident during her own training came to her mind. The individual had not been a close friend, but Dr. Singer suddenly and vividly recalled her shock, her peers' reactions, and the department's handling of the incident. Dr. Singer's thoughts then went to her own son, soon to graduate medical school. She cringed internally at the idea that this could happen to him or one of his peers. Her personal experience helped guide the tone of her questions. No personal information was disclosed, but the empathic setting Dr. Singer could provide may have helped Tammy, at this point, to spontaneously talk about her friend and how she killed herself. Rebecca jumped from the roof of the main adult inpatient hospital building. Tammy learned about the death at a Pediatrics Department emergency meeting. She attended Rebecca's funeral and spoke with her family. In a state of disbelief, at times close to tears but unable to cry, Tammy talked about their friendship. Dr. Singer learned that in spite of feeling lonely, since her friend's suicide, Tammy had been experiencing a decreased interest in socializing, especially with friends of Rebecca's, "Rebecca was the person I would turn to." She had initially avoided walking in front of the building from which her friend jumped, but was now able to walk there in the company of someone. While she remained less engaged with the world, her appetite and energy, which had significantly decreased after her friend's suicide, were improving. She reported experiencing moments of deep sadness at the thought of her friend, alternating with anger. Frequently, she found herself imagining what it would be like to contemplate the thought of jumping from a building. She imagined what it must have been like for her friend. She imagined the jump itself. At careful assessment she denied suicidal ideation.

Principles of Diagnosis and Management

Diagnosis

Dr. Singer considered posttraumatic stress disorder (PTSD) and adjustment disorder with depressed mood as the most likely diagnoses. Tammy's clinical presentation met most criteria for PTSD, which is characterized by a combination of intrusion symptoms, avoidance, and changes in thinking, mood, and arousal ([1]; see Chap. 5 for further discussion and for Chap. 5, *Table 5.1: Posttraumatic Stress Disorder: Core Features*). She had been exposed to a traumatic event, the violent death of a close friend. She experienced partial avoidance of cues related to the traumatic event, such as exposure to mutual friends, and being in spatial proximity to the place where her friend had died. It was later learned that Tammy had skipped work a few times in the 2 weeks after the incident. Though she was entertaining the thought of quitting her professional training, with effort she could now go to work every day. Noticeably she was able to talk about her deceased friend and the circumstances of her death with a level of distress proportionate to the circumstance. Overall avoidance symptoms had been worse immediately after the trauma occurred, but were improving by the time she met Dr. Singer. Tammy also experienced changes in her mood and thinking and a variable extent of anger and guilt. She experienced decreased interest in social activities, felt a sense of detachment, and her overall ability to enjoy life was diminished. Tammy also demonstrated changes in arousal, including poor concentration, hypervigilance at work, and intermittent initial insomnia. She denied having intrusion symptoms (such as distressing memories, dissociative symptoms, and intense physiological reactions to reminders of the trauma), hallmarks of PTSD, with the exception of a couple of anxious dreams in which a patient on her service was not responding to treatment for high fever, both of which occurred after she had forgotten to write an order for a patient. Considering the lack of recurring intrusion symptoms, and variable severity and persistence of other symptom categories, Dr. Singer favored the diagnosis of adjustment disorder with depressed mood, given the presence of a recent stressor associated with distress and impairment in her full functioning, while not meeting full criteria for PTSD. The differential diagnosis further included the syndrome of complicated grief after bereavement, a common manifestation after the unexpected and violent death of a close relative or friend to suicide [2, 3]. Tammy had not experienced the pathognomonic persistent and disruptive yearning for the deceased, and difficulty accepting the death, which characterize the syndrome of complicated grief. The lack of enduring sad mood or anhedonia differentiated her state from a typical major depressive episode, though age of onset and most other symptoms made this diagnosis one to consider. The temporal association to a traumatic event, short duration, and quality of the anxiety she experienced, intermixed with angry and sad mood, did not support a diagnosis of generalized anxiety or another anxiety disorder.

Management and Treatment

The choice of treatment for adjustment disorder depends on the symptom constellation, character traits, coping style, psychosocial history and life circumstances at the time the disorder ensues, the initial impression about which treatment modality the patient may best respond to, and the patient's preference. Supportive psychotherapy aims to support and enhance the patient's already existing constructive coping mechanisms to help adaptation to life circumstances perceived as stressful. In cognitive behavioral psychotherapy, cognitive distortions and maladaptive beliefs, such as the ones which develop during an adjustment disorder or PTSD, are reframed and corrected; graded exposure to fear-evoking stimuli is a behavioral strategy used to treat avoidance symptoms related to traumatic exposure. Interpersonal psychotherapy can be applied to the treatment of symptomatology related to problems in interpersonal arenas, including grief over loss and role transitions, both of which pertained to Tammy's presentation, in addition to interpersonal disputes and interpersonal skill deficits. Psychodynamic psychotherapy can be indicated in treating adjustment disorders when the patient's symptoms and maladaptive coping mechanisms, in response to specific life circumstances, appear motivated by thoughts and feelings out of the patient's awareness and usually related to past life experiences. Central to this psychotherapeutic modality is the attention given to the transference developed in the therapeutic relationship as a vehicle for change.

The addition of medication, including anxiolytics, antidepressants, and sedative-hypnotics, may be helpful in the treatment of adjustment disorders and PTSD for symptom relief in selected cases. Careful screening for a substance use disorder and attention to increasing use of and dependence on sedative-hypnotics/anxiolytics are essential in the management of patients experiencing symptoms of PTSD.

Principles for Doctors Treating Doctors

During her assessment, Dr. Singer had learned that following the death of Tammy's middle brother, the entire family entered psychotherapy with a family therapist. In Tammy's recollection, her mother was the main focus in the treatment, as she may have been clinically depressed. Her mother had suffered earlier from postpartum depression after the birth of the same brother, when Tammy was 3 years old. Dr. Singer considered that circumstances around the loss of her brother might have contributed to the development of Tammy's rigid and controlling character traits. The history suggested that these traits intensified around times of separation, such as during adolescence and first year of college, leading to restrictive eating, compulsive exercise, and a tendency to emphatically avoid depending on others for help. Dr. Singer recognized that the same traits may also have functioned as a strength, contributing to Tammy's high achievements both as a student and competitive dancer, and to her motivation to become a pediatrician in light of her brother's doctors' inability to save him. Dr. Singer anticipated that Tammy's fierce independence and controlling attitude could initially interfere with the establishment of a therapeutic alliance and effective response to psychotherapy, but in the end would also be an asset to Tammy's recovery.

At the end of her assessment, Dr. Singer had a set of aims in mind. Tammy's mood and her neurovegetative and cognitive symptoms needed to rapidly improve so that she could resume baseline social and occupational functioning and continue to safely work as a doctor in training caring for patients. She needed to be monitored for the higher risk of suicide typically encountered in survivors of suicide victims [4], and also observed as a phenomenon related to the influence of suggestion on suicidal behavior, leading to the so-called imitative suicide [5]. In addition, she needed to grieve the loss of her friend and revisit the mourning of the loss of her brother to prevent the development of symptomatology akin to her reaction to her friend's suicide when exposed to future medical catastrophes and encounters with death in her career as a physician. Tammy's belabored decision to become a physician was once more challenged by her friend's suicide, which she could not help but blame on the imagined failure of the medical establishment to keep her friend alive. She eventually needed help to recognize that her current anger was reactionary to the powerlessness she felt once more about not being able to save a loved one and, additionally, it was a displacement of anger at her friend for having abandoned her. Fundamental to Tammy's development as a healthcare provider was relinquishing the wish to be able to prevent all medical calamities, not only in her loved ones but also in her patients. Hand in hand with this process, she needed to regain confidence in herself, her training hospital, and the discipline of medicine. She needed to be able to continue to work as ambitiously as she had set out to do while developing awareness of, and tolerance for, the realistic limitations of the medical profession.

The main challenges Dr. Singer foresaw, in beginning treatment, included Tammy's anger and undermined trust in healthcare providers, including her own psychiatrist, and the survivor's guilt she might have experienced in relation to the death of her friend and the earlier death of her brother, now projected as blame toward her training institution. Dr. Singer's initial therapeutic approach included risk management, psychoeducation, supportive measures, the use of cognitive behavioral strategies, and medication. She explained to Tammy that her symptoms were secondary to her exposure to a traumatic event and were possibly further aggravated by its resemblance to her childhood loss. Tammy's higher risk for suicidal ideation and behavior and the need for monitoring were addressed directly. Aware that lack of social support is the largest single predictor of developing PTSD after a traumatic event [6], Dr. Singer encouraged Tammy to reach out to supportive figures in her life and have as much contact as feasible with friends and family. Tammy was instructed to continue to expose herself in a graded manner to reminders of the traumatic event, initially in the company of other people and eventually on her own. Sleep hygiene measures and the brief use of sedative-hypnotics were recommended to normalize her sleeping patterns. Concerned about Tammy's ability to sustain a regular workload under the circumstances and to facilitate rapid recovery, Dr. Singer suggested a course of sertraline, a serotonin reuptake inhibitor, commonly indicated for the treatment of mood and anxiety disorders and PTSD. Tammy took this advice skeptically. After doing her own research, she accepted a prescription for trazodone, a sedating antidepressant that is not a sedative-hypnotic, which she chose to use on an as-needed basis for insomnia while reserving the decision about other medications to a later time.

While Tammy attended her twice-weekly appointments regularly, she was often 5–10 minutes late. Her demeanor was somewhat distant and controlling. Her descriptions of symptoms and personal experiences were packaged in psychological jargon. At times she brought in articles about treatment strategies Dr. Singer had recommended and posed challenging questions as if responding to the need to be one up on Dr. Singer and prove her wrong and inadequate. This behavior allowed her to reveal little about herself and progress seemed slow to Dr. Singer. At this point, Dr. Singer thought that psychodynamic psychotherapy may be a better suited treatment modality. It would offer the opportunity to explore Tammy's reactions to the therapeutic relationship, which seemed to interfere with her getting the help she needed, and explore the impact her childhood loss may have had on her recent reaction to the friend's suicide. Dr. Singer focused on Tammy's behavior in the sessions: "Are you wondering whether I know enough to be able to help you?" Tammy tuned in and replied, "Rebecca's doctor was not able to help her...I guess I should not assume that you are all the same. It's hard to do that. I have seen enough failures in my life." Slightly puzzled and with a half-smile of recognition and relief on her face, she recalled that after her brother died, her parents were quite skeptical of doctors, would do their own "research" themselves prior to doctors' visits, also brought in articles with scientific information, and sought second opinions when a family member had a concerning medical problem. When asked, Tammy recalled wondering whether her parents could have done more to get her brother the care he needed, but was very uncomfortable with that thought and never asked them. In this context she remembered a couple of disturbing dreams, representing different versions of herself or other doctors not being able to help a patient, or getting stuck in repeated failed attempts to provide care to a patient. "It must be hard not knowing whether you can trust yourself, me, or your other role models to do a good job, after the failures you have witnessed," Dr. Singer replied. As Tammy's anger and anxiety about trusting others and herself were addressed in relation to her past experience and her relationship with Dr. Singer, she started showing more spontaneous affect and connecting with Dr. Singer in her sessions. Over 3 months, Tammy's symptoms and functioning improved. Later in the year, during a busy rotation, she started missing appointments, rationalizing this by way of a busy schedule, and explaining, "my patients are a lot sicker than I am, I don't know that I need to be here much longer." Noticing her comparison to her sicker patients, Dr. Singer interpreted Tammy's avoidance of help, coinciding with her improvement, as related to unconscious guilt about having survived her brother and her friend: "It seems that it is difficult to see yourself get better while neither your friend nor your brother had that chance." This line of interpretation helped Tammy stay enough on track with her treatment and opened the way to addressing her ongoing difficulty accepting help from others.

As Tammy's anger at the medical establishment started dissipating, awareness of sadness about the loss of her friend seeped in. She was able to contemplate other explanations for Rebecca's death, including severe depression, rather than failures on someone else's part. She wondered less whether she could have done something more to prevent the death and recalled fun memories of vacation trips she and her friend shared while in training together. Now Tammy was ready to acknowledge having felt belittled and rejected by her friend's suicide and to see how she had displaced her anger onto others and herself. She was steadily more connected with friends and participating in social life. As her relationship with Rebecca was becoming articulated into a complex narrative, Tammy could elaborate about the loss of her brother as a separate experience and even start exploring her guilt about resenting him as the cause of her mother's depressive episodes when he was born and when he passed away. Importantly, this step in her treatment helped Tammy not continue to experience future calamities as a mere repetition of her childhood trauma. This meant that she was on her way to develop the flexibility to use a larger and more constructive repertoire of coping skills, other than externalization, withdrawal, and rigidity, in response to negative outcomes to be encountered in her profession.

While a third-year resident, and during a rotation in the pediatric emergency department (ED), Tammy woke up one night with a panic attack. She felt she could not breathe and had palpitations and an acute sense of fear. She assumed this was a panic attack, took deep breaths, and recovered in about 15 minutes from acute anxiety. The day before, she had assessed an adolescent girl in the ED for a suicide attempt, 3 months after she had discharged the same girl from the ED for superficial wrist cutting, under recommendation of the ED psychiatric consultation service. Tammy's anxiety about her career choice resurfaced: "This job is impossible. No matter how hard you try, something is bound to go wrong." Tammy now wondered whether she should take medication and expressed doubts about Dr. Singer's ability to help her, saying, "I'm not sure you've helped me enough – I guess I need meds for that." In the context of a relapse of symptoms, Tammy expressed renewed ambivalence about getting help. Dr. Singer understood Tammy's panic attack as a sign of regression related to her overall progress. Under exposure to a reminder of previous traumas, the fear of separation from her caretaker in the setting of her improvement and maturation as a physician mobilized anxiety, as it had previously occurred during similar developmental transitions. Tammy's unconscious conflict about her wish to be taken care of, which had earlier led to the development of a rigid and independent character style, continued to be worked through, and new solutions to the conflict became accessible. Throughout their treatment, Dr. Singer used both her understanding of the mind and psychodynamic principles and her shared experiences of being a physician – including the development of the physician role, the experience of being a trainee in a hierarchical hospital system, and the aspirations of serving patients and gaining mastery over the ever-expanding field of medicine.

Outcome

Tammy reencountered various versions of her struggles during the continuation of her treatment with Dr. Singer, which lasted until the end of her training. Particularly troubling was Tammy's rotation through a pediatric oncology service, where for the first time a patient of hers died while under her care. These experiences gave her a chance to work through her main developmental struggles and residual effects of the traumatic losses of her life, including anxiety about separation, conflict around depending on others, difficulty trusting physicians and herself as capable, and guilt about having survived loved ones. Relying on the coping skills which had supported her success throughout her development, Tammy joined a residents' wellness group that just formed in her institution. In a shared social environment, she learned more about coping with the challenges of her profession and felt less isolated in her experience. Within the group she initiated a mentorship program for medical students on stress management during medical training and later developed an interest in ethical aspects of medical decision-making, which remained an area of focus after completion of her residency. Tammy knew that she may again have difficulty coping with anger and anxiety in reaction to the powerlessness she was bound to encounter from time to time in her medical career and in her life and felt less shameful and more open to the prospect of seeking help again.

Pearls
- Survivors of suicide victims are at higher risk of suicide and need careful and ongoing monitoring. The risk may be heightened in peers sharing affiliation with the suicide victim.
- Lack of social support is the largest single predictor of developing PTSD after a traumatic event.

- Physicians are prone to personally take charge of medication recommendations and regimens prescribed by their treating physician. This behavior can undermine the efficacy of their treatment, and it should be tactfully addressed.
- For a variety of motivations, physicians may be at risk of using the rationalization that their patients are sicker or needier than they are, to avoid taking care of their health as seriously as they take care of their patients.
- A course of psychotherapy may be helpful when a previous experience of trauma, especially if attributable to a medical calamity, is suspected to be negatively influencing a physician's coping style.

References

1. American Psychiatric Association. Diagnostic and statistical manual of mental disorders. 5th ed. Arlington: American Psychiatric Publishing; 2013.
2. Hawton K. Complicated grief after bereavement. BMJ. 2007;334:962.
3. Mitchell AM, Kim Y, Prigerson HG, Mortimer-Stephens M. Complicated grief in suicide survivors. Crisis. 2004;25(1):12–8.
4. Bartik W, Maple M, Edwards H, Keirnan M. The psychological impact of losing a friend to suicide. Australas Psychiatry. 2013;21(6):545–9.
5. Stack S. Media coverage as a risk factor in suicide. J Epidemiol Community Health. 2003;57:238–40.
6. Brown CR, Andrews B, Valentine JD. Meta-analysis of risk factors for post-traumatic stress disorder in trauma-exposed adults. J Consult Clin Psychol. 2000;68:748–66.

Suggested Reading

Beck JS. Cognitive behavior therapy: basics and beyond. 2nd ed. New York: Guilford Press; 2011.

Jordan JR. Is suicide bereavement different? A reassessment of the literature. Suicide Life Threat Behav. 2001;31:91–102.

Markowitz JC, Petkova E, Neria Y, et al. Is exposure necessary? A randomized clinical trial of interpersonal therapy for PTSD. Am J Psychiatry. 2015;172:430.

Shelder J. The efficacy of psychodynamic psychotherapy. Am Psychol. 2010;65:98.

Winston A, Pinsker H, McCullogh L. A review of supportive psychotherapy. Hosp Community Psychiatry. 1986;37:1105.

Chapter 10
The Case of Ruth Daughtery: Navigating Catastrophic Illness in a Family Member

Anna L. Dickerman

Case

Ruth, a 32-year-old internal medicine attending at a teaching hospital, presents to Dr. Nuer, a local psychiatrist in private practice who is her contemporary, with the chief complaint: "I just have a lot of stress right now." Ruth, who has never seen a psychiatrist before, quickly defends her decision to seek care, stating "I'm not crazy, I just need some help working through things." Dr. Nuer cannot help but notice that Ruth appears fatigued and on the verge of tears as soon as she sat down in the office. Ruth quickly and matter-of-factly reveals that her mother, with whom she has a close relationship, is being treated for metastatic lung cancer at a prestigious oncology facility, getting "the best care possible." Her mother has already gone through surgery and several rounds of chemotherapy, and her prognosis is poor. Ruth surmises aloud

A. L. Dickerman, MD (✉)
Weill Cornell Medical College/New York-Presbyterian Hospital,
New York, NY, USA
e-mail: and2033@med.cornell.edu

© Springer Nature Switzerland AG 2019 115
J. S. Gordon-Elliott, A. H. Rosen (eds.), *Early Career Physician Mental Health and Wellness*,
https://doi.org/10.1007/978-3-030-10952-3_10

that her mother probably has less than a year to live as she rattles off data from recent publications about her mother's diagnosis. As Ruth speaks, Dr. Nuer finds herself struggling to keep up with her notetaking and becoming drawn in by the medical details. Ruth shares that in addition to traveling over an hour each day back and forth to see her mother in the hospital, she is in contact with her mother's treatment team throughout the day – getting updates so that she can "make sure I keep an eye on what's going on over there." Because of this, Ruth has been struggling to finish her own patient care and administrative duties in a timely fashion and getting little sleep in the process. She breaks down in Dr. Nuer's office and describes to Dr. Nuer feelings of intense guilt about being a "terrible daughter and even worse doctor." As the only physician in her family, she feels pressured to oversee her mother's care and experiences anxiety whenever she is unable to do so. She is resentful toward her family but ashamed of this resentment. She wishes she could just spend "quality time" with her mother but feels unable to do so. Her patients and colleagues noticed that she seems tired and distracted. She asks Dr. Nuer if it might be worth considering taking a leave of absence from her position at the hospital, though she is concerned she could be perceived as "weak" or "dumping work" on others. Aside from her situationally decreased sleep, Ruth denies any neurovegetative signs or symptoms. She feels she has no time to participate in enjoyable activities given her situation but that she "would love" to be able to go to the gym and spend more time with her friends. She denies suicidal ideation or use of any mood-altering substances.

Principles of Diagnosis and Management

Diagnosis

The most appropriate diagnosis for Ruth is adjustment disorder with anxiety. Adjustment disorders are stressor-related illnesses in which patients suffer from intense distress and/or impairment of functioning. DSM-5 defines these disorders as "the presence of emotional or behavioral symptoms in response to an identifiable stressor(s) occurring with 3 months of the onset of the stressor(s)" [1]. Adjustment disorders do not include normal bereavement or exacerbation of pre-existing mental health conditions, and symptoms must subside within 6 months of the removal of the stressor. Six sub-types of adjustment disorders exist: depressed mood, anxiety, mixed depressed mood and anxiety, disturbance of conduct, mixed disturbance of emotions and conduct, and unspecified. Dr. Nuer's differential for Ruth includes major depressive disorder, anxiety disorder (generalized anxiety disorder and obsessive compulsive disorder), acute stress disorder (ASD) and post-traumatic stress disorders (PTSD), and cluster C personality disorders. What ultimately helps Dr. Nuer in coming to her diagnosis is the clear new onset of symptoms in the setting of a specific major life event. In contrast to a major depressive episode, Ruth is not experiencing core symptoms of anhedonia nor any neurovegetative changes. Unlike primary anxiety disorders, Ruth has not ever experienced debilitating anxiety prior to her mother's illness. Her intact relationships and interpersonal function make the diagnosis of a personality disorder less likely. Finally, Ruth does not endorse the characteristic symptom clusters of increased arousal, avoidance, and intrusion that are key to making the diagnosis of ASD or PTSD.

Management and Treatment

The mainstay of treatment for adjustment disorders is psychotherapy. Pharmacotherapy is not typically indicated, though judicious use of targeted and time-limited medication such as PRN benzodiazepines for anxiety/insomnia can be useful in some cases where patients' symptoms are severe enough to impediment to daily functioning. Psychotherapeutic approaches to adjustment disorders are often supportive in nature, with a focus on crisis intervention, problem-solving, and education. Though there is a lack of controlled clinical trials of specific psychotherapy modalities, both interpersonal psychotherapy and brief psychodynamic psychotherapy are felt to be reasonable approaches [2–4], as are behavioral interventions [5].

Principles for Doctors Treating Doctors

Illness in a relative or loved one can be particularly challenging for physicians. An important theme which often arises in the treatment of such individuals is difficulty with the role transition from physician to family member [6]. The physician-relative may become overinvolved in the medical management, which can in turn compromise care and pose problems for all involved parties. Indeed, Ruth has begun to feel burdened by her family. She feels trapped by the expectations of her family but also fearful of disappointing her colleagues. Chen and colleagues outlined four sets of competing and often conflicting expectations that can cause distress among doctors with an ill family member, including internal standards of being the ideal physician vs. ideal family member and external pressures from family members and other physicians [7]. Ruth is struggling with these conflicts and is only able to engage with her ill mother from the standpoint of a physician, attempting to direct her medical care rather than spending "quality time" together. One of Dr. Nuer's challenges in treating Ruth will be to help her navigate these role conflicts and gain greater flexibility in her ability to care for her mother not only as a physician but also as her daughter. As she begins to explore how Ruth would most want to spend meaningful time together at the end of her mother's life, this may be met with some resistance, in part due to the fact that anxiety in physician-patients often leads to denial of symptoms or their meaning. In Ruth's case, she notably does not dwell on the topic of her mother's prognosis, instead using an intellectualized approach which becomes infectious at times for Dr. Nuer. By throwing herself into the medical details of her mother's disease, Ruth may be warding off the painful reality of impending loss. There may also be an unconscious need to feel omnipotent [8], which makes it difficult for the doctor to acknowledge her own vulnerability or inability to save a loved one. The physician with a sick family member is undoubtedly frightened, though he or she may have difficulty admitting this. Indeed, Ruth minimizes her psychic distress to Dr. Nuer almost immediately. Due to these factors, Ruth will likely do well in treatment with a dynamically oriented but supportive approach that fosters and protects the therapeutic alliance while maximizing adaptive coping strategies [9]. The question of whether to take time off from work is one which is likely to cause angst for many physicians. Doctors rarely take sick leave and often work when they themselves feel unwell; medical training often places a value on compulsiveness which can lead to guilt or an exaggerated sense of responsibility [10]. Sometimes, as is true for Ruth, there is an underlying fear that asking for help signifies weakness [11, 12]. Dr. Nuer needs to be aware of these apprehensions as she helps Ruth navigate her difficult situation and make the decision most likely to best serve her own mental health and well-being. Common countertransference reactions that Dr. Nuer may experience include anxiety and overidentification. Her proximity in age to Ruth may make her particularly vulnerable to the latter, which can be problematic in treatment [13]. As a physician herself, Dr. Nuer may be able to provide a positive and healthy role model for identification. Judicious and mindful self-disclosure, where appropriate, may help decrease some of Ruth's shame and facilitate exploration of more painful or anxiety-provoking material.

Outcome

Ruth meets with Dr. Nuer for once weekly psychotherapy over the next several months. She is gradually able to extract herself from her mother's medical care, checking in with the oncologists once weekly as opposed to daily. When she visits her mother, she spends time with her watching their favorite movies and listening to music together, as opposed to discussing the next steps in her treatment. Ruth feels progressively less burdened by her family and her mother's illness but continues to struggle with balancing her competing responsibilities at the hospital. After considering the pros and cons with Dr. Nuer, she decides to apply for family medical leave. She struggles with shameful feelings related to taking time off from work but ultimately feels relief in being able to focus on her family's needs during this difficult time. As her mother's condition worsens and the reality of her mother's prognosis becomes more difficult to avoid, Ruth experiences a spike in anxiety and depressed mood. Dr. Nuer focuses the therapeutic work at this point on anticipatory bereavement. She helps guide Ruth in identifying goals for finding meaning at the end of her mother's life and imagining what life will be like after her death. Ruth continues to work with Dr. Nuer for several months after her mother's death as she transitions back to full-time work at the hospital. By approximately 6 months after her mother's death, she continues to experience intermittent feelings of sadness when she thinks about her mother but has maintained intact occupational and social function.

Pearls
- Adjustment disorders are stressor-related illnesses characterized by intense distress and/or impairment of functioning that subsides within 6 months of the removal of the stressor. Psychotherapy, often supportive in nature, is the mainstay of treatment.
- Illness in a relative or loved one can be challenging for physicians. The role transition from doctor to family member is often met with anxiety. Common defense mechanisms seen in these cases include denial and intellectualization.
- Physicians also often struggle with balancing the potentially competing interests of the needs of their colleagues and patients with those of their own men-

tal health and well-being. When indications for a leave of absence arise, doctors may struggle with feelings of guilt and shame about this.
• Overidentification is a common reaction experienced by the treating physician in such cases and is best handled with mindful use of psychotherapeutic techniques which foster therapeutic alliance while also helping the patient maximize adaptive coping.

References

1. American Psychiatric Association. Diagnostic and statistical manual of mental disorders. 5th ed. Arlington: American Psychiatric Publishing; 2013.
2. Carta MG, Balestrieri M, Murru A, Hardoy MC. Adjustment disorder: epidemiology, diagnosis and treatment. Clin Pract Epidemiol Ment Health. 2009;5:15.
3. Maina G, Forner F, Bogetto F. Randomized controlled trial comparing brief dynamic and supportive therapy with waiting list condition in minor depressive disorders. Psychother Psychosom. 2005;74(1):43–50.
4. Markowitz JC, Kocsis JH, Fishman B, Spielman LA, Jacobsberg LB, Frances AJ, Klerman GL, Perry SW. Treatment of depressive symptoms in human immunodeficiency virus-positive patients. Arch Gen Psychiatry. 1998;55(5):452–7.
5. Van der Klink JJL, Blonk RWB, et al. Reducing long term sickness absence by an activating intervention in adjustment disorders: a cluster randomized controlled design. Occup Environ Med. 2003;60:429–37.
6. Schneck S. "Doctoring" doctors and their families. JAMA. 1998;280:2039–42.
7. Chen FM, Feudtner C, Rhodes LA, Green LA. Role conflicts of physicians and their family members: rules but no rulebook. West J Med. 2001;175(4):236–9.
8. Ellard J. The disease of being a doctor. Med J Aust. 1974;2:318–23.

9. Misch DA. Basic strategies of dynamic supportive therapy. J Psychother Pract Res. 2000;9(4):173–89.
10. Gabbard GO. The role of compulsiveness in the normal physician. JAMA. 1985;254:2926–9.
11. Vaillant GE, Sobowale NC, McArthur C. Some psychologic vulnerabilities of physicians. N Engl J Med. 1972;287:372–5.
12. Waring EM. Psychiatric illness in physicians: a review. Compr Psychiatry. 1974;15:519–30.
13. Meissner WW, Wohlauer P. Treatment problems of the hospitalized physician. Int J Psychoanal Psychother. 1978–1979;7:437–67.

Chapter 11
The Case of Bianca Cring: Professional Loyalty and Personal Infidelity

Elena Friedman

Case

Bianca, a 30-year-old fourth-year surgery resident at a big academic medical center, came to see Dr. Hamon, a young female psychiatrist, with the chief complaint: "I don't know what I am doing, I am messing up my marriage." Bianca presented as bright, affable, and well put together. She arrived 5 minutes late, for her initial evaluation, apologizing profusely. She seemed ashamed to be in Dr. Hamon's office and explained that she had never seen a psychiatrist before and felt unsure of where to begin. Despite her initial unease, Bianca presented as well related and quickly opened up about her childhood, current life, and the events prompting her visit.

Born and raised in a midsized college town on the West Coast, Bianca is the only child of two successful physicians. They both took particular pride in their work. Growing up,

E. Friedman, MD (✉)
Weill Cornell Medical College/New York-Presbyterian Hospital, New York, NY, USA
e-mail: elk2013@med.cornell.edu

© Springer Nature Switzerland AG 2019   123
J. S. Gordon-Elliott, A. H. Rosen (eds.), *Early Career Physician Mental Health and Wellness*,
https://doi.org/10.1007/978-3-030-10952-3_11

Bianca was fascinated by her parents' jobs; she played with toy stethoscopes and proclaimed that she too was going to become a doctor. During her teenage years, Bianca questioned her wish to become a doctor. She felt frustrated with her parents' demanding work schedules and at times felt envious of the attention they bestowed upon their patients. She wondered if this was a future that she wanted for herself. Bianca initially denied any history of depression to Dr. Hamon; however, as she elaborated on her experience, it became clear that Bianca suffered from a depressive episode during high school. She described feeling conflicted about her career trajectory, feeling sad and anxious on a daily basis, not sleeping well, a loss of appetite with a resultant 15 pound weight loss, isolating herself from social experiences, and did not even look forward to activities – such as going to the movies or hiking – which she once enjoyed. Bianca remembered feeling tired all of the time. Nonetheless, she threw herself into her work with a particularly intense focus on SAT prep and getting into a top college. She attributed her symptoms to the "stress" of high school and found that by her senior year, once accepted to her first choice school, her symptoms abated. In the months leading up to college, Bianca decided that she wanted to become a doctor after all and entered college as a premed. In college, Bianca had another depressive episode following the end of a long-term relationship. Her boyfriend, who graduated 2 years ahead of her, broke up with her after he started dating someone else. Bianca was devastated and confused but again threw herself into her work, concentrated on getting into medical school, and felt better within a few months. She got into a top medical school and eventually matched into her first choice residency program. She prided herself on being hardworking, dependable, and having very close relationships with her colleagues.

During her fourth year of medical school, Bianca met her now husband. She was instantly attracted to him. He was witty, sociable, and handsome. He worked in finance, lived nearby, and traveled often for work. She had a lot of free time to spend with him during her fourth year of medical school, and their relationship quickly became serious. She felt comfortable with him and his family, and he seamlessly connected to her friends. To Bianca, it seemed as if their lives were intertwined already. They got married 2 years later, and a year after that, she gave birth to a baby boy Xavier.

Bianca had a difficult time bonding with Xavier. She felt very anxious and guilty that she did not produce enough breast milk to feed Xavier but also hated the expectations that she had to feed him every meal. She felt demoralized and futile as a mother and entertained thoughts that perhaps her husband and son would be better off if she were dead. This was the first time in her life she had suicidal thoughts. Bianca did not share this with anyone. She avoided friends and family for weeks. She did not seek treatment and felt ashamed that she was a bad mother. Bianca responded to her experience by returning to residency at 8 weeks postpartum instead of the 12 weeks she planned to take off. Returning to work was a relief for Bianca.

When Bianca came to see Dr. Hamon, Xavier was 11 months old. Bianca stated that she did not feel depressed. She was sleeping well and keeping up at work. She no longer had suicidal thoughts. She reported that she and her husband were arguing more in recent months, as he felt that she should work less and spend more time with their son. She felt that he did not understand or respect the nature and requirements of her surgery residency. She did not even want to share with him that her department chair already invited her to stay on as faculty at the academic center after graduating residency. She felt well respected and valued within her department and wanted to stay. Her husband, however, was frustrated with her plans, stating that he had expected her to work part time and tend to their family. Their interactions were regularly contentious. She felt misunderstood and undervalued as a partner and focused her time and energy on building collegial relationships with her co-residents. With one co-resident in particular, she felt a particular connection. They started to spend more time together, and several months after her return from maternity leave, they began an intimate relationship. She felt most at ease at work and was spending progressively less time at home. She felt confused and worried about the future of her marriage.

Principles of Diagnosis and Management

Diagnosis

Bianca's chief complaint involved cheating on her husband with a co-resident and concerns related to the future of her marriage. It is important to note that this behavior may or may not be related to a specific psychiatric diagnosis. In some cases, cheating could be a symptom or a result of a psychiatric disorder. In other cases, it may be a manifestation of the patient's relationship dynamics and internal conflicts.

Dr. Hamon suspected that Bianca suffered from recurrent major depressive disorder with an episode during high school, college, and most recently, following her son's birth. The prevalence of postpartum depression in the general population ranges from 6.5% to 12.9% [1]. Previous depressive episodes as well as limited partner support and marital difficulties are significant risk factors for development of postpartum depression. Postpartum depression is associated with increased risk of marital conflict and impaired infant-caregiver attachment [1].

In addition to major depressive disorder (MDD), Dr. Hamon's differential for Bianca's presentation included bipolar disorder and a substance use disorder. Bianca's depressed mood, poor sleep, concentration difficulties, and low mood could have contributed to her decision-making in the above scenario. Negative, ruminative thinking and difficulties bonding with her husband, both symptoms of depression, could have exaggerated her experience of disconnect from her husband. Manic symptoms, such as inflated self-esteem, increase in goal-directed activity, lack of sleep, hypersexuality, and impulsivity, could have been part of the clinical picture that contributed to Bianca's infidelity. Abusing substances impairs one's judgment and leads to decisions that one may not have made if they were sober.

When Bianca presented to Dr. Hamon, she no longer met criteria for a major depressive episode. She enjoyed working and spending time with her son. She felt anxious about her marriage but did not feel sad or hopeless. She denied symptoms of insomnia, change in her level of energy or appetite. She was not manic and denied current or past substance abuse. In summary, while the confluence of new parenthood and a depressive episode likely impacted her marriage, this does not fully explain the circumstances prompting her evaluation with Dr. Hamon. Her current feelings and behavior were likely part of an internal conflict and the struggle to make healthy interpersonal and career decisions.

Management and Treatment

The mainstay of treatment for depression, and specifically postpartum depression, is psychotherapy with or without medication management, based on the severity of the symptoms. Therapies that can be helpful include supportive psychotherapy, psychodynamic psychotherapy, cognitive behavioral therapy, and interpersonal psychotherapy. Serotonin reuptake inhibitors (SRIs) are most commonly used alone or in combination with psychotherapy for moderate to severe depression. Since Bianca no longer fit the criteria for a major depressive episode, she did not require an SRI. Bianca's psychiatric history however necessitates close monitoring for recurrence of symptoms. Previous depressive episodes are a risk factor for future depressive episodes. Dr. Hamon recommended that Bianca begin psychotherapy utilizing a range of supportive, psychodynamic, and cognitive behavioral techniques in order to help her understand the conflict within her marriage as well as within herself. Couples therapy may also be helpful though Bianca initially declined this recommendation.

Principles for Doctors Treating Doctors

Upon presentation, Bianca denied a history of depression or anxiety. However, with careful attention to early life experiences, Dr. Hamon hypothesized that Bianca's postpartum depression several months prior to her presentation was her third lifetime depressive episode. Notably, all episodes were untreated. Though Bianca is a physician and learned about major depressive disorder during her medical training, she failed to recognize it in herself, demonstrating a lack of self-awareness when it came to her own symptoms and internalized stigma related to psychiatric illness and treatment. During young adulthood, Bianca recalled feeling unable to manage her feelings and sadness but was ashamed that she may need help. Her physician parents cared for sick people; she did not want to add to their burden. Bianca believed that seeing a psychiatrist was an admission of weakness and could inhibit her chance to become a physician herself. She thought of her parents who worked tirelessly without complaints. On occasion, she overheard them discuss colleagues, who expressed feeling overwhelmed and depressed. Their responses were always this person was "not cut out for this kind of work." Feelings and difficulty managing one's emotions were signs of weakness that inhibited one's ability to practice medicine. If Bianca could not manage "feeling sad," how could she manage medical school, residency, and life as an attending. To her mind, minimizing her experience was the most appropriate course of action. As her parents dedicated themselves to their work, frequently at the expense of tending to their family, Bianca too attempted to address her depressive symptoms with increased focus on her academics. Studying and work seemed like a logical self-directed treatment for her mood episodes. This patterned repeated itself. When she had doubts about her career, she studied more. When she felt sad about a breakup, she spent more hours at the library. When she felt inadequate as a mother, she went back to work to reconnect with an experience of competency. Medicine provided Bianca with a sense of identity and meaning; it also served as a mechanism of avoidance and denial. It is worth noting that Bianca experienced her capacity to "push through" as synonymous with her success rather than an awareness that her hard work, dedication, and intelligence led to her position in a competitive residency.

The long hours and significant demands of physician training can influence the development and/or exacerbation of depression and prevent one from seeking treatment. The demands of training can also distract one from thinking about and working through internal conflicts and relationship difficulties. Bianca did not seek treatment to address her difficulties bonding with her son and her husband. Instead she reflexively went back to work. Developing a close relationship with a co-worker was an extension of her usual pattern of delving into work to avoid problems at home. She did not seek treatment to try to work through her feelings; instead, she acted on them by having an affair. Bianca found it easier to discuss a specific behavior: infidelity, rather than feelings of sadness and disappointment.

In many medical specialties, during training, physicians must work long hours and have little control over their schedules. Time with family is limited and hard to predict. It can be difficult for non-physicians to appreciate this, and as a result, colleagues are apt to form strong friendships that often begin out of an appreciation for each other's day-to-day experiences. Physicians in specialties like surgery are at a higher risk for divorce than physicians in other specialties [2]. One study found that female physicians had a higher divorce rate (37%) than their male colleagues. Physicians who reported themselves to be less emotionally close to their parents also had a higher divorce rate [2]. Another study found that female physicians who reported working more than 40 hours per week had a higher probability of divorce than those working fewer hours per week [3]. Bianca's experience includes all these risk factors.

Bianca scheduled to meet weekly with Dr. Hamon but regularly missed sessions due to work. She did not want to ask for time off for her own care and often felt that she was

not worthy of treatment and that her problems were insignifi-
cant. She oscillated between feeling guilty about her affair
and justified that she was connecting to a person who
admired and respected her. Initially, Dr. Hamon overidenti-
fied with Bianca, as she too could feel misunderstood by her
non-physician husband. She colluded with Bianca's stance of
"us (physicians) against them (non-physicians)" and empathized with Bianca's wish to build intimate relationships with
others who appreciated her dedication to medicine. Dr.
Hamon minimized the impact that Bianca's actions could
have on her family. She neglected to explore Bianca's frequent absences. Dr. Hamon colluded with Bianca's lifelong
pattern of idealizing her medical career and dismissing much
else. With time however, Dr. Hamon became increasingly
frustrated with Bianca's regular absences and dismissal of
their work together. Within the therapeutic frame, Dr.
Hamon experienced both Bianca's dynamic with her co-
worker (two physicians working in the trenches together,
lamenting about others, who don't understand their field) and
Bianca's dynamic with her husband (being angry and frustrated about the person's dismissal of her work). Dr. Hamon
used her own discordant feelings about Bianca to understand
and to bring to the surface Bianca's internal conflicts. She
explored Bianca's dedication and idealization of medicine as
well as her anger at her husband. In order to succeed in treatment, Bianca needed to address her conflicts and feelings
rather than increase her attention to work. She had to accept
the role of the patient and commit to receiving help. Assigning
importance to therapy, something other than her career, was
the first step to valuing her feelings and her life outside of
work.

Outcome

Bianca continued to see Dr. Hamon weekly and soon started
attending sessions bi-weekly. She initially highlighted her
admiration of her parents' work ethic though with time, she

was also able to access her anger toward them for seemingly prioritizing their patients above their family. Gradually, she expressed sadness and disappointment that her parents were rarely available. She discussed her fears of repeating this pattern with her own son. Bianca began to appreciate that having feelings or needing and asking for help were both normal and important. She began to discuss her anger at and disappointment with her husband. Working through her feelings lessened her need to act them out, and she eventually ended her relationship with her co-resident. She and her husband started couples' therapy. Bianca focused her energy into self-awareness and awareness of those around her. To her enormous surprise, engaging in treatment did not impede upon her professional successes but led to gains in her life outside of work.

Pearls
- Significant demands of physician training, including long hours, unpredictability, and the emotionally difficult nature of the work, can influence the development and/or exacerbation of depression and can prevent one from obtaining treatment in a timely fashion.
- Depression and symptoms of depression, such as poor sleep, general lack of interest, hopelessness, negative thinking, and difficulty bonding, can lead to poor decision-making, lack of care about consequences of one's actions, and feelings of being disconnected from one's partner. All of these could increase the likelihood of infidelity.
- Physicians in especially demanding specialties, such as surgery, are at a higher risk for divorce than physicians in other specialties. Female physicians, especially those working more than 40 hours per week, have a higher probability of divorce. Physicians who report less emotional closeness to their parents also have a higher divorce rate.

- Physicians treating physicians have to take great care not to overidentify with their patients and not to minimize their patients' career and interpersonal difficulties. A neutral provider can empathize not only with her patient's identity as a physician but with other aspects of the patient's life and identity as well. Neutrality can help the physician explore how the patient's specific dynamics surrounding career and work affect the patient's relationships.
- Becoming conscious of and processing internal conflicts can help stop maladaptive thoughts and behavior patterns.

References

1. Steward D, Vigod S. Postpartum depression. N Engl J Med. 2016;375:2177–86.
2. Rollman B, Mead L, Wang N-Y, Klag M. Medical specialty and the incidence of divorce. N Engl J Med. 1997;336:800–3.
3. Ly A, Seabury S, Jena A. Divorce among physicians and other healthcare professionals in the United States: analysis of census survey data. BMJ. 2015;350:h706.

Chapter 12
The Case of Anita Rao: Defining a Career and a Self

Bernadine H. Han

Case

Anita Rao is a 31-year-old internal medicine resident in her second postgraduate year at an academic medical center in New England. She requested treatment through her hospital's house staff wellness and mental health program and was referred to Dr. Lee, a senior psychiatrist on the hospital faculty, with the chief complaint of "I don't know what to do with my life!" Anita was on time for her appointment, friendly, and a little anxious, articulating herself well and with humor; she was easy to like. She shared that she found herself "stressed" and losing sleep over making a decision about the next step in her career path. She was a strong resident in her program, well-respected by her peers and her attendings, and always received positive feedback in her rotations. She had a meeting with her program director about a month ago to discuss career planning and has since felt torn about what she should do after residency. She had always imagined a career committed to underserved primary care, possibly in geriatrics, but

B. H. Han, MD, MS (✉)
New York University School of Medicine/Bellevue Hospital
Center, New York, NY, USA
e-mail: bernadine.han@nyumc.org

© Springer Nature Switzerland AG 2019   133
J. S. Gordon-Elliott, A. H. Rosen (eds.), *Early Career
Physician Mental Health and Wellness*,
https://doi.org/10.1007/978-3-030-10952-3_12

she was now also considering a fellowship in pulmonology and was flattered by the encouragement from her attendings to submit case reports and present at conferences. With fellowship deadlines looming, she was becoming more anxious about contacting references and preparing her applications. As she expected, she had loved her outpatient rotations and the specialness of "being someone's doctor," but she was also surprised to find how much she enjoyed the fast-paced nature of critical care in the intensive care unit (ICU). She had good hands for tricky procedures, and she found satisfaction in the concrete application of the physiology she had been learning since medical school while on the unit. Outside of work, she had become engaged to her boyfriend, whom she had been dating since medical school. While she always thought of herself as someone with modest tastes and a low appetite for luxury, planning for a wedding and future family has begun to make her think about income maximization, schedule flexibility, and financial planning in a new way.

Making career decisions has always felt hard for Anita; she took time off after college (where she majored in English literature with a minor in studio art) before enrolling in a premedical program to complete her science prerequisites. She was a bit of a romantic and felt pulled by the humanities and social justice initiatives in college and medical school. She knew she was an idealist and felt she should be guided by her morals, though she sometimes wondered if that got in the way of knowing what she wanted. Anita was the youngest of three daughters, and her oldest sister Sheela's example as a wife, mother, and highly accomplished academic cardiologist eventually inspired her to be, like Sheela, a woman who could "have it all." Anita also liked the feeling that Sheela was pleased by and proud of her pursuit of medicine, and Anita tried to remember interesting cases or EKGs that she could talk about when they saw each other. In medical school, Anita performed better than average academically and developed close relationships with peers. At the same time, she found her clinical rotations challenging because she often overly connected to her patients, which could make her feel she was on the "wrong team." She felt that some of her residents were impatient with the time she spent with or the extra questions she asked her patients. She sensed that they more consistently prized efficiency, objectivity, and even a kind of jaded distance in clinical care more than her efforts to make a real connection. Her current dilemma reminded her of this experience in medical school, and she worried that her enjoyment of the ICU suggested that she was not as compassionate toward her patients as she imagined.

She stated, "I know everyone else is trying to figure out their careers, too, but I don't know why it feels harder for me!" She complained of difficulty falling asleep for the last month, specifically because she ruminated about various career trajectories. She acknowledged being "a lifelong planner" but lately found herself more preoccupied with dates, deadlines, and perhaps more generalized worry, finding that she had no appetite some days. Over the last month, she even had a handful of crying bouts, overwhelmed by the extremes of her options and fearful that she will feel either understimulated but faithful to her ideals in the clinic or engaged, but fraudulent and possibly overstressed, in a critical care unit. Getting back into a regular running schedule and doing yoga a few times a week were helpful, but her symptoms persisted. She continued to do well on the wards and enjoyed her time with her fiancé and her friends. It was helpful to either "vent or just get my mind off things."

Anita was never hospitalized or suicidal. She spent about a year in weekly therapy for anxiety before starting college. She also saw a psychiatrist who prescribed escitalopram 10 mg for generalized anxiety disorder at the end of college, and this was continued without change by her primary care provider in the years since. During both treatment episodes, Anita experienced significant anxiety in the context of transitions (high school and college graduations) that led to fear and catastrophizing thoughts about leaving home and college, respectively. Anita drank "a cocktail or two" with friends on Saturdays and sometimes a glass of wine with dinner during the week. She smoked marijuana "socially, maybe every couple months," stating that she likes how both substances helped her relieve a little stress but felt it would be irresponsible to use them more than she does now.

Principles of Diagnosis and Treatment

Diagnosis

The best working diagnosis for Anita's current presentation would be adjustment disorder with anxious features. Adjustment disorders are characterized by the onset of emotional or behavioral symptoms following a specific identified stressor. These symptoms must develop within 3 months of the stressor, and they must cause notable distress and/or impairment that is beyond what might be expected by the nature of the stressor. Following a career planning meeting last month, Anita started to experience anxiety with disruptive changes to her sleep and appetite, though her ability to function in her professional and personal life appeared intact. She continued to exhibit good concentration and energy at work and other activities and continued to find pleasure in her job and her social life. Her anxiety stems specifically from an impending decision about choosing a fellowship and career path. Though her anxiety may bring her down at times, she does not have the persistent feelings of sadness or anhedonia that would suggest a major depressive disorder. She was previously diagnosed with generalized anxiety disorder (GAD), which was treated with a year of psychotherapy and for which she continues to take an SRI. The most important diagnosis on the differential is a relapse of GAD, and this should be carefully considered. Dr. Lee should continually monitor Anita for signs that her anxiety is becoming more generalized, severe, or impairing. At the time of her initial evaluation with Dr. Lee, the development of Anita's anxiety in the specific context of a perceived increase in pressure on career and fellowship decisions and the lack of this severe anxiety when thinking about or doing other things (including while at work, at play, or spending time with her loved ones) more strongly suggests an adjustment disorder. Anita would likely not be experiencing her symptoms if she were not currently approaching this unique career-defining decision. She does have a historical pattern of experiencing stress and anxiety during similar times, and this likely increases her vulnerability to greater distress during this time. She does not describe symptoms consistent with panic disorder, phobia, trauma-related disorders, or obsessional-compulsive disorders, though all of these should be at least briefly considered in a patient who presents with anxiety.

Her substance use does not appear to be significant enough to create prominent use-related anxiety or other symptoms, though potential effects of intoxication or withdrawal from alcohol, marijuana, and other substances should remain in Dr. Lee's mind, particularly if further history suggests prior heavier use followed by a decrease or discontinuation in use over recent weeks to months. Cannabis and alcohol can both increase insomnia, anxiety, and depression in acute and extended withdrawal syndromes.

Anita described long-standing psychological conflicts related to difficulty with the separation and individuation of early adulthood that appear to be activated in her current situation. Closely related to these conflicts are a personality style characterized by a strong motivation to please and a reification of ideals. These traits have clearly contributed to her likability in social and professional situations, her successful journey through medical training thus far, and her clinical empathy with patients. They also appear to cloud Anita's ability to assess reliably what drives and inspires her in the absence of having someone to please.

Management and Treatment

Adjustment disorders are most commonly treated with psychotherapy, though medications may be useful in cases where symptoms (and stressors) are persistent and severe. In Anita's case, Dr. Lee may reasonably think about an increase in her dose of escitalopram, especially if Anita's anxiety worsens or persists, and there is a good chance that she will notice benefit from the increased dose. There may be more than one appropriate and effective psychotherapeutic modality, particularly in a patient like Anita, who engages easily in a positive therapeutic relationship. She would likely feel benefited by supportive, cognitive-behavioral, and psychodynamic approaches or an eclectic approach informed by all three. Because of her previous experience with psychotherapy, Anita may be open to returning to treatment, and her initial evaluation suggests that she has capacity and curiosity for introspection and self-reflection. Anita may find adequate relief from her anxiety with a relatively short course of weekly treatment, less than or up to a year. If she wishes to continue beyond this, she may find usefulness in psychotherapy for the remainder of her residency training, particularly as she follows through with her eventual decision and transitions to her next career step. Like many medical trainees, Anita has prominent obsessional character traits in a neurotic personality organization. Her personality style and structure clearly play a role in the various contributory conflicts that she described in her initial presentation, as well as in the anxiety she currently experiences. Psychotherapy will highlight her strong inclinations to please others and maintain certain high ideals, as well as the effect of these motivations on her behaviors and difficulties in making choices.

Anita is certainly not the only resident in her peer group experiencing anxiety about her career decision-making. Some training programs may offer opportunities for peer support in the form of process groups or moderated wellness programs, and if available, these may also provide a forum to facilitate a sense of being both understood and part of a community [2].

Principles for Doctors Treating Doctors

From the earliest stages of medical training, there are multiple points at which identity is broken down and redefined or refined, re-creating a kind of professional adolescence and formalized stages of career-defining separation/individuation. While it is common in many fields to make career decisions throughout one's working life, medical training ritualizes and universalizes these differentiating decisions in such a way that they must be anticipated and planned for, perhaps long before trainees feel ready for or convinced of their choices. Whether choosing a residency, a fellowship, a job, or a career setting, the trainee (and even the fully formed physician) must renounce all other possibilities, often before knowing the nature of all their options. These decisions may be complicated by the pressure of being one of a large cohort of peers making their decisions concurrently, all guided by different motivations and markers of success, and creating a perception (and perhaps reality) of competition that may further influence one's choice. These career-defining choices are often greeted with joy and conviction, but they also frequently involve a degree of mourning for the road not taken, particularly if the choice was a difficult one. Of course, the trainees' decisions are subject to uncontrollable forces, including the National Resident Matching Program (i.e., "the match") and the local job market for a chosen specialty. A good fit for a given trainee may depend as much on a specialty's lifestyle and subculture as on the trainee's enjoyment of the discipline itself. Financial and geographic factors (which in turn affect proximity to social and family supports) may also grow increasingly important with advancement through the developmental stages of adulthood, including marriage, child-rearing, and care of aging parents. Whether because of the internal pressures of the field or the external enticements beyond it, at every point in the journey toward and of physicianhood, students, trainees, and full-fledged doctors may face a decision to leave the field altogether. The goodness of the decision's fit among an array of variables directly affects the trainee's sense of wellness and thus their potential for burnout. Multiple factors contribute to the future doctor's sense of purpose both in work and in life beyond work, and maximizing this sense of purpose can maximize wellness and minimize burnout.

From the beginning of medical training, and perhaps even earlier, a student/trainee begins to develop a meaningful sense of self as a physician. This new identity of the trainee emerges in new roles, interacting with patients, peers, attendings, and other medical staff in new settings, with new purpose. Crossing the threshold of medical school demands that students break their previously held social norms and boundaries as they shift from laypeople to clinicians – to ask intimate questions of strangers, to reveal and examine another's anatomy, and to cut skin with a blade. Forging and integrating this new doctor's identity into one that most likely was already (or nearly) fully formed can be powerful and destabilizing on a trainee's sense of self. Both unexpected disappointments and pleasant surprises along the way to becoming a fully practicing doctor may be disruptive to the trainee's professional identity formation and can elicit a range of intense emotions, including loss, fear, rage, and pride. As such, the process is difficult per se, and it can be made worse with the necessary developmental step of resolving the trainee's projected ideals of self and career with reality. The field of medicine itself is attached to a particular shared narrative of identity formation that often involves a journey of inspiration, struggle (long hours, difficult exams, deprivation of sleep, food, or other basic needs), challenges, and achievements. This narrative highlights pride in some of the medicine's core values: "self-sacrifice, duty, hierarchy, ability to perform competently in adverse circumstances" [1]. These values may be in direct conflict with those of an individual trainee, and this conflict may cause the trainee, the training directors, or both to feel compromised.

All of Anita's peers are grappling with their own decision-making processes, with or without similar degrees of anxiety. It goes without saying that the rigors and demands of training may result in a variety of stress-related psychiatric symptoms, and trainees with different biological vulnerabilities, personality styles, or psychological structures may well manifest this stress with more significant mood, cognitive, or behavioral symptoms. Anita's history of previous treatment and benefit from care likely minimized her hurdles in accessing mental health care as her distress increased. Most of her peers will turn to their friends, family, or mentors for guidance. It is interesting to consider how Dr. Lee's approach to Anita might differ if she were his mentee and not his patient. In either case, Dr. Lee may strive to facilitate Anita's ability to assess her own values and goals with greater clarity. Students and trainees may be hesitant to see a psychiatrist during their training, particularly if they have not previously had good experiences, or any kind of experience, in mental health treatment. Fear of being pathologized, stigmatized, or "analyzed" may delay or prevent trainees from seeking appropriate evaluation or care. Anxiety around appearing dependent, needy, or weak in the therapeutic relationship may present a challenge to the trainee's ability to utilize treatment. Despite assurances of confidentiality, the trainee may also be uncomfortable in treatment with someone who might be in a position of evaluating student or house staff performance or who may be close to those who would. As someone well indoctrinated into the norms and structure of medicine, Dr. Lee may easily forget or minimize both the position of vulnerability that students and trainees occupy in the medical hierarchy and the stigma that psychiatric or psychological treatment still carries in the medical world. Acknowledging the trainee's concern about being a patient in the same system in which he or she is also a provider may be an important validation in building trust and rapport.

Dr. Lee may well be able to empathize with Anita's situation, and his identification may be useful in the treatment. Overidentification, of course, can cause its own difficulties, including a lack of curiosity or an avoidance of the uncomfortable position of the trainee [3]. There may be a temptation to be self-disclosing of one's own experience, and of course, there may or may not be benefit to sharing. This temptation itself may be a manifestation of a need or idealization active in the transference, which may result in Anita's disappointment when unindulged. In this and other ways, the countertransference may offer rich information about Anita's difficulties. Feelings of pride or flattery or urges to advise or warn may reflect Anita's own wishes to be pleasing, idealizing, or taken care of. In the transference, Anita may feel parented, or she may long for a friend; she may be fearful of evaluation or appear overly deferential before a respected faculty member. The nature and duration of treatment may variously determine the appropriateness of pointed transference analysis, though even without an intensive analysis, the transference may illustrate the object relations that make Anita's decision so difficult. Remaining attuned to these pulls in the countertransference can help Dr. Lee express empathy for Anita's unconscious conflicts while avoiding an enactment, particularly one in which Dr. Lee becomes another person whom Anita is hoping to make proud. Achieving this can facilitate a holding and neutral space where Anita can feel safe to explore the anxieties and pressures affecting her ability to make a decision.

Outcome

Anita agreed to meet with Dr. Lee in weekly therapy. They discussed in the first few weeks whether they should trial an increase in Anita's escitalopram, though they decided not to make the change as Anita noted feeling better within the first month of weekly meetings. They discussed Anita's experience throughout her life as the youngest in a family with impressive accomplishments, and while she always felt that her family showed interest and support in her activities, she always felt like the baby, not quite taken seriously. She developed a habit of trying to find ways to "live up to" everyone else in her family and perhaps people outside her family. She said, with some surprise, "It's like every new attending on every new rotation became someone else to impress!" She recognized that in her efforts to please others, she also put herself in the position of feeling guilty when she did not choose them or their interests for herself. "I guess I've trapped myself," she observed. She was able to find connection to the work and interactions that provided her with a sense of meaning, namely, a feeling of pride in her ability to care about and be moved by the human side of illness, even in the ICU where her patients were often easily turned into a set of vital signs and lab values. Over the course of a few months, Anita began to prepare applications for a fellowship in palliative care. Now in the fall of her final year of residency, Anita submitted her fellowship rank list to the match, which will take place in the next couple months. She is happy that she will continue to have combination of inpatient and outpatient work, and she describes a sense of privilege in being present during such significant times in the lives of her patients and their families. Anita's anxiety continues to be well-managed even as she makes plans for her wedding the following summer and her sleep and appetite recovered quickly. Anita acknowledged a mild increase in her anxiety in anticipation of the match results, and she plans on continuing therapy through the end of residency, jokingly commenting, "Who knows what else will stress me out once I start thinking about leaving here!"

Pearls
- Medical training involves an induction into a new culture, which demands the forging of a new professional identity.
- Professional identity formation may be a joyous or painful process, but it often involves conflict and potential mourning of the forced disavowals of still wished-for career options.
- Mental health professionals who treat students and trainees are in a unique position to connect the trainee to a sense of self-appreciation and value while empathizing with the sacrifices and small losses of self that the training environment demands.

References

1. Roberts LW, Warner TD, Lyketsos C, Frank E, Ganzini L, Carter D, Collaborative Research Group on Medical Student Health. Perceptions of academic vulnerability associated with personal illness: a study of 1,027 students at nine medical schools. Compr Psychiatry. 2001;42:1–15.
2. Kahn NB Jr, Schaeffer H. A process group approach to stress reduction and personal growth in a family practice residency program. J Fam Pract. 1981;12(6):1043–8.
3. Lane LW, Lane G, Schiedermayer DL, Spiro JH, Siegler M. Caring for medical students as patients. Arch Intern Med. 1990;150:2249–53.

Suggested Reading

Cohen MJM, Kay A, Youakim JM, Balacius JM. Identity transformation in medical students. Am J Psychoanal. 2009;69:43–52.

Frost HD, Regehr G. "I AM a Doctor": negotiating the discourses of standardization and diversity in professional identity construction. Acad Med. 2013;88:1570–7.

Gentile JP, Roman B. Medical student mental health services: psychiatrists treating medical students. Psychiatry. 2009;6:38–45.

Goldie J. The formation of professional identity in medical students: considerations for educators. Med Teach. 2012;34:e641–8.

Holden M, Buck E, Clark M, Szauter K, Trumble J. Professional identity formation in medical education: the convergence of multiple domains. HEC Forum. 2012;24:245–55.

Wilson I, Corwin LS, Johnson M, Young H. Professional identity in medical students: pedagogical challenges to medical education. Teach Learn Med. 2013;25:369–73.

Chapter 13
The Case of Regan Cooper: Anxiety in a Gay Resident

David Hankins and Gwen L. Zornberg

Case

Regan is a 27-year-old first-year psychiatry resident who presented to Dr. Wood, a psychiatrist working in the resident mental health program, with the chief complaint of "I'm feeling anxious." Regan reported 2 months ago experiencing a brief and intense period of anxiety (marked by sudden sweating, shortness of breath, and an intense feeling of imminent danger) during a departmental grand rounds presentation. Initially, Regan could not clearly recall the sequence of events leading to this episode, but after discussing it on the telephone with close friends back home, she came to realize that the precursor was a statement made by a senior faculty member during the subsequent question period about the "demonstrated benefit" of conversion therapy for homosexuality as "good practice that can cure the problem"; Regan recalled being "jarred to attention" at this moment, followed by the described rush of "fight or flight" symptoms.

D. Hankins, MD, MEd · G. L. Zornberg, MD, MSc, ScD (✉)
Weill Cornell Medical College/New York-Presbyterian Hospital, New York, NY, USA
e-mail: dgh7001@nyp.org; glz9002@med.cornell.edu

© Springer Nature Switzerland AG 2019   145
J. S. Gordon-Elliott, A. H. Rosen (eds.), *Early Career Physician Mental Health and Wellness*,
https://doi.org/10.1007/978-3-030-10952-3_13

Dr. Wood asked Regan to elaborate more on that event in the lecture hall. Regan went on to say that, raised in a progressive community and educated in largely liberal urban environments, she has felt affirmed as a gay woman. Before this comment by the senior faculty member, she had not been specifically attuned to examples of mean-spirited comments directed at her or other LGBTQI (gay, lesbian, bisexual, transgender, queer, and/or intersex) individuals during her medical training. She reported feeling supported by the administration of both her medical school and residency. After some reflection, however, a number of subtle examples of bias or discrimination came to mind. She recalled being asked about her "boyfriend" by a supervising attending. And at the beginning of intern year, an older male patient had commented jokingly, but clearly disapprovingly, on Regan's hairstyle, which she wore short, saying that a "pretty young woman" might want to have "longer hair in order to meet a husband." Upon reflection, Regan noted to Dr. Wood that these events felt linked in her memory.

Over the session, Dr. Wood learned that Regan grew up with her mother, father, and two brothers in a diverse West Coast city where Regan fit in well and enjoyed having many close friends. In residency now at a Midwestern medical center, Regan had so far been a high-performing and well-liked resident. She described not yet feeling she had an "established" group of friends in her new environment, but she made sure to keep in regular contact with friends from home and medical school and was making efforts to meet new people. She had not dated much since high school and had been sexually active very selectively, attributing this to a strong focus on values, clinical academic achievement, and research pursuits – "I've always had so much on my plate, and I have high standards." She was interested in having a partner "to share my life with" in the future.

Regan described feelings to Dr. Wood of being taken aback that anyone could be discussing gay conversion therapy as a current practice, moreover as a "standard of care." She began to realize that it had felt like a personal attack and stirred up images of reports of a couple of recent news events involving hate crimes. A few days after the episode at the grand rounds talk, Regan, who continued to feel "rattled" even after getting support in phone conversations from friends back home, tried to talk about what had happened with a co-resident whom she believed to be gay, thinking he might be "a good place to start" – as a peer and someone who had also heard the comment about conversion therapy. Regan disclosed to him her thoughts about the senior faculty endorsing "cruel, maybe even barbaric" treatment, and the classmate responded quizzically and not particularly supportively. Regan recalled feeling doubly appalled and more "alone" at that moment – a feeling that seemed to linger for several days.

On psychiatric review of symptoms, Regan endorsed the short-lasting anxiety symptoms during the grand rounds discussion. These symptoms had not recurred, and she did not particularly find herself worried that these might occur. She reported "a couple of sleepless nights" after the lecture and also recalled a few days after the incident of finding it more challenging to focus at work as intensively as usual. Since then Regan's self-reported mood returned to being "mostly pretty happy." She had no hopelessness or wishes for life to end nor any history of depression, past suicidality, or a problematic substance use. A sense of "lack of connection" with others at work had remained. She admitted that, since this event, she had been – for the first time – "aware" of being gay in a community that was much less inclusive than what she had previously experienced. She was starting to "observe" subtle, and sometimes not so subtle, negative attitudes and bias. She looked for resources or initiatives in diversity at her institution and was coming up with few leads. She found herself starting to doubt her choice for residency training to move out of the community where she had felt comfortable prior to residency. She realized that she had felt protected from much of this discrimination before now. She told Dr. Wood that she didn't like feeling the way she had felt briefly. She wanted to be comfortable during the time spent in her new community or at least make this a positive 4 years.

Principles of Diagnosis and Management

Diagnosis

One of the first questions that Dr. Wood considered in the assessment was whether Regan's symptoms met criteria for a DSM-5 diagnosis. The most appropriate diagnosis for Regan's new onset of anxiety and negative mood related to experiences of being confronted with critical ideas about, and responses to, being gay (the senior lecturer's comments about conversion therapy and the dismissive co-resident) is adjustment disorder with mixed anxiety and depression. The brief moments during that grand rounds of surging of anxiety with diaphoresis, palpitations, and fear of dying are suggestive of a panic attack. Nonetheless, Regan did not report anticipating, or avoiding, having additional episodes like this; hence DSM-5 diagnostic criteria for panic disorder were not met. Similarly, Regan experienced a few days of low mood coupled with insomnia, but that did not meet full criteria for a major depressive episode, and there were no lifetime symptoms of a manic episode. Other anxiety disorders, such as generalized anxiety disorder, could be explored; in the absence of more enduring anxiety symptoms, emotional and physiologic, this is less likely. Aware of the increased risk among LGBTQI and other minority populations of alcohol and other substance use disorders, Dr. Wood noted to herself that in the initial differential diagnosis, the brief anxiety episode could have represented symptoms related to any one of several substance use disorders or withdrawal from substances, but this did not fit with Regan's reports of minimal alcohol use and no other substance use.

As she continued to formulate her thoughts about Regan, Dr. Wood reflected more on the use of psychiatric diagnoses in the setting of minorities, including individuals who are gay or bisexual like Regan. While LGBTQI identity is most appropriately viewed as a cultural factor, much like racial identity, and not cause for a psychiatric diagnosis, there is a long and fraught history of psychiatric assumptions regarding LGBTQI psychosexual development [1]. In the absence of any scientific evidence, homosexuality was classified as a mental disorder (perversion) in earlier editions of the DSM (eliminated in 1973), warranting treatment [2].

Lastly, Dr. Wood considered whether, in fact, Regan met criteria for any psychiatric diagnosis and considered an alternate perspective of Regan's anxiety as an expectable expressed response to Regan's experience of prejudice. This experience of discrimination raised her first serious concerns about her chosen geographical location for residency training as the best place to establish a profession career and personal life.

Management and Treatment

Individuals diagnosed with a DSM-5 diagnosis of adjustment disorder are usually treated with psychotherapy; medications may be considered in certain circumstances. Cognitive behavioral therapy (CBT) could be implemented with a focus on identifying and exploring thoughts and feelings triggered by situations, including interpersonal encounters, cultural messages, or one's own automatic beliefs about oneself and the world. With CBT techniques, Dr. Wood could assist Regan in more clearly and objectively identifying how subtle microaggressions or more blatant negative messages and experiences that confront or devalue a person's sense of identity may lead to negative emotions and self-beliefs when ubiquitous and sustained. Interpersonal skills could be developed to help Regan feel more equipped to express herself and respond assertively to challenges in her environment – with the goal of enhancing her sense of empowerment and resilience. Supportive psychotherapy and psychodynamically informed psychotherapies could be used to assist Regan in more exploration of her experiences and how they fit into other areas of her overall identity – enhancing her integrated experience of self and her connection with others.

Should Regan's symptoms worsen rather than resolve, a serotonin reuptake inhibitor (SRI) may be the first-line pharmacologic approach to reduce symptoms of anxiety and depression. The sexual side effects of SRI-based antidepressants are important to counsel patients about and to monitor for during the course of treatment. Even a brief trial of a benzodiazepine or another sedative-hypnotic anxiolytic; risks, including cognitive dulling, anterograde amnesia, and/or the potential for escalating use, which may render such agents problematic, hence they should be used with caution.

LGBTQI individuals, as members of minorities that experience widespread prejudice, are reported to be at elevated risk for suicide. Safety should be assessed continually over the course of treatment.

Principles for Doctors Treating Doctors

One of the challenges in addressing the mental health and wellness needs of the gay resident arises before the person presents for evaluation, namely, the individual may not even seek care. The usual factors that lead to delay and avoidance of receiving treatment common to all residents, such as cost and time, may apply to the gay resident, who also faces obstacles specific to gay identity; these include, but are not limited to, concerns of bias impacting the evaluation and treatment – based on psychiatric conceptions of non-conforming sexuality that were not based on scientific evidence. Negative attitudes, limited knowledge and awareness of gay individuals and issues, and frank anti-homosexual bias and discrimination remain pervasive. LGBTQI-identified residents have limited spaces that support their safe inclusion [3]. Some may seek mental health treatment with hope of finding a venue for self-expression in a nonjudgmental therapeutic relationship, while others may avoid such treatment out of concern that prejudice may be even more significant in the mental health setting. Decades following removal of homosexuality as a DSM diagnosis, anti-homosexual attitudes have remained in the practice of mental healthcare [1]. To date, there are psychiatrists who adhere to the belief that nonconforming sexuality is a perversion and some who still attempt to conduct "conversion" therapies of LGBTQI individuals. Someone like Regan might delay or avoid seeking care due to skepticism about being able to find a therapist who is not only "tolerant" but truly able to address issues specific to her integrated identity and be wholly supportive and affirming of who she is [4].

Once the trainee has sought care, additional issues specific to LGBTQI-identified patients differentiate their treatment from that of those from other groups, including other minority groups. Depending on the particular reasons the patient came for help and the presence of any psychiatric disorders, the treatment may focus on areas of self-identity, belonging, discrimination, and other complex psychological and interpersonal matters. For a patient like Regan, as in most cases, there will be a combination of issues that are related to being gay and those that are not so tightly connected to these experiences. At her stage of training and life, Regan may be seeking enhancement of integrating an identity as a professional psychiatrist with comfortable expression of being openly gay, as well as general adaptation into adulthood and physicianhood. The gay physician in training may also be grappling with bias or other explicit or implicit messages that arise in their work with colleagues and patients. Regan might find that she wants to explore in therapy how to think about – and address, when needed – the way in which patients' projected ideas and attitudes about her as a gay person will influence the doctor-patient relationship and treatment and the psychological impact of this on her. The isolation she is feeling in her new environment can be validated. As a gay resident, securing a sense of affiliation with a critical mass of individuals who form a common bond of shared experiences can prove even more challenging to achieve while immersed in the demands of a residency program; more difficult, moreover, in a less inclusive community than one has previously experienced. A resident like Regan may be concerned about marginalization during her career due to elements of her identity, particularly where there is a dearth of similar people. This is more stressful when the individual feels that it is a matter of survival to hide one's real identity [5]. This remains an issue in the academic medical field, in which the barriers to entry and advancement of LGBTQI people may remain [3].

The clinician will want to be attentive to the various issues that may emerge in the treatment and to do so while demonstrating a supportive and affirming stance. As a general guide, clinicians without substantial experience in working with LGBTQI-identified patients should strongly consider seeking additional supervision or training to enhance attitudes and knowledge relevant to the treatment they are beginning. One example of a misstep that an inexperienced or uneasy clinician might make is to minimize or miss the impact of the patient's experience of living as an underrepresented minority. A patient's concerns about being judged or discriminated against may lead the clinician to experience the patient as "paranoid," while such concerns may represent a reasonable response to a personal history of never belonging or fitting in, depending on factors in the person's environment and the person's psychology. On the other hand, the clinician may be overly focused on the LGBTQI identity, missing pertinent aspects of the history not related to sexual identity and development or unnecessarily reducing the patient's troubles as somehow all connected to their experience as a gay person. Such assumptions may lead to misdiagnosis and mistreatment. Additionally, they may seriously damage the therapeutic relationship and potentially make the patient wary of seeking psychiatric care in the future.

Discomfort based on lack of experience leading to uneasiness, tentativeness, or – conversely – overconfidence may lead the clinician to have difficulty building rapport and gaining the trust of the gay trainee. Concerns about how the clinician's limited experience might impact the therapeutic encounter will not uncommonly arise explicitly, with the patient actively seeking out clinicians who are skilled in helping gay individuals and who are openly gay, themselves. The patient may have questions for the therapist about previous knowledge of, or exposure to, LGBTQI issues. The psychiatrist's own concerns about inadequacy or inexperience may prompt tensions between anonymity and disclosure; additionally, they may provoke countertransference responses, such as feeling deskilled, judged, or exposed – potentially leading to problematic unconscious responses, from prematurely referring the patient to another clinician, to being overly zealous in the treatment, to avoiding supervision out of concerns for having one's "inexperience be seen." Asking therapists to reflect on their own heteronormative assumptions is crucial to ensuring that gay people are treated equally to their counterparts.

Outcome

After three sessions of history gathering and initial exploration, Dr. Wood reflected back to Regan that there have been specific psychiatric symptoms (the panic attack and then a period of anxiety and mood disturbance) which would be worth monitoring – especially given the potential for future exposure to microaggressions in the context of the stressors of residency. Dr. Wood also commented that there were other issues about Regan's sense of fitting in to her new residency training community in a very different part of the country and about her professional future that seemed highly relevant to her right now, and which could be explored further. For this, Dr. Wood suggested starting weekly therapy, and Regan, relieved by the opportunity for a space to talk about these things and feeling a positive connection with Dr. Wood, happily agreed. Dr. Wood sought supervision from a colleague who had joined the faculty with more clinical experience and knowledge of diverse LGBTQI issues and experiences. Dr. Wood felt fortunate to have direct access to a colleague with such experience, knowing that many clinicians do not.

Over the course of treatment, Regan's comfort with Dr. Wood grew, and she adopted a generally positive transference. She began to talk more about her sense of self within the context of sexual identity. Dr. Wood validated Regan's experiences and realistic concerns about the anti-gay messages prominent in society while also affirming Regan's capacity to form and strengthen her own professional identity as a psychiatrist and continue to live a life that is meaningful, productive, and successful. With respect to Regan's experience and future as a physician, Dr. Wood utilized their common identities as physicians to help Regan internalize the belief that it requires strength and skill to thrive on the margins of many cultures and in a profession where LGBTQI identities are not necessarily always supported or even tolerated – whether through direct messaging in the profession, society at large, or by internal processes, for example, internalized homophobia [6]. Six months into treatment, Regan was beginning to speak with more clarity about her responses to aggression and was able to find a few gay peers to affiliate with in and out of the medical center. During one session, Regan mentioned an idea she had to approach her graduate medical education administration about developing educational programming and supports for LGBTQI residents at the hospital. While Regan expressed to Dr. Wood that she knew that her initial motivation for wanting to do this was a desire to feel involved and "connected" as she had during medical school and earlier in life, she also believed that this would be a meaningful way to try to contribute to her professional community at a systems level. The development of a health curriculum inclusive of issues pertaining to LGBTQI individuals, and fostering a medical culture that is empowered to address personal and institutional homophobia through education and training, will help to create a workforce that can navigate issues relevant to the LGBTQI community; such efforts enhance patient care and the professional growth and personal well-being of clinicians [3].

Near the end of Regan's third year of residency, Dr. Wood accepted a new job in a town a few hours away. She offered Regan referrals to continue her treatment, but Regan – after further discussion – decided she felt "ready" to end the therapy.

They worked on the loss of their relationship during their termination phase and reflected on the work they had done together. Their treatment ended at the same time Regan was submitting applications for fellowship, which she hoped to do in the institution where she had attended medical school. Regan felt grateful for the opportunities she experienced during residency but knowing that returning to a more developed, inclusive environment would be better for her, personally and professionally. The LGBTQI inclusive educational initiatives she had helped to create continued after her departure, and over the next 10 years of her career, she was invited back on an annual basis to be part of a week of hospital-wide diversity programming.

Pearls
- LGBTQI-affirmative therapy requires knowledge, skills, and attitudes relevant to the LGBTQI-identified person's experience. Supervision, expert consultation, or appropriate referral should always be considered.
- Gay identity may be considered a cultural factor, not a diagnosis. Being gay should not be assumed to be contributing to an individual's psychological difficulties.
- LGBTQI doctors considering psychotherapy may hesitate to engage or remain in therapy, as an array of negative theories of nonconforming sexuality have pervaded the clinical discourse and practice of psychiatry over the past century. This has had profoundly harmful effects on LGBTQI people and their families.
- Thoughtfully implemented psychotherapy can assist gay trainees to enhance resilience during residency training and professional growth.

References

1. Committee on Human Sexuality: Group for the Advancement of Psychiatry. In: Drescher J, editor. GAP monograph: homosexuality and the mental health professions: the impact of bias. Hillsdale: The Analytic Press; 2000.
2. Drescher J. Out of DSM: depathologizing homosexuality. Behav Sci. 2015;5(4):565–75.
3. Sánchez NF, Rankin S, Callahan E, Ng H, Holaday L, McIntosh K, Poll-Hunter N, Sánchez JP. LGBT trainee and health professional perspectives on academic careers--Facilitators and challenges. LGBT Health. 2015;2(4):346–56.
4. King M. Attitudes of therapists and other health professionals towards their LGB patients. Int Rev Psychiatry. 2015;27:396–404.
5. Mansh M, White W, Gee-Tong L, Lunn MR, Obedin-Maliver J, Stewart L, Goldsmith E, Brenman S, Tran E, Wells M, Fetterman D, Garcia G. Sexual and gender minority identity disclosure during undergraduate medical education: "In the closet" in medical school. Acad Med. 2015;90(5):634–44.
6. Erickson-Schroth L, Glaeser E. The role of resilience and resilience characteristics in health promotion. In: Eckstrand K, Potter J, editors. Trauma, resilience, and health promotion in LGBT patients. Cham: Springer International Publishing; 2017.

Chapter 14
The Case of Katherine Moss: Caring for Oneself to Care for Others

Anna Salajegheh

Case

Katherine Moss, a 38-year-old psychiatrist, recently finished fellowship at the hospital at which she is currently an attending. Her chief complaint at initial evaluation was: "I'm finding it hard to focus on my work since I've finished cancer treatment." She was referred to Dr. Blake by a former supervisor.

At her initial appointment, Katherine, who was 10 minutes late, smiled sheepishly and offered Dr. Blake a cookie, saying she had walked by one of her favorite bakeries on the way to her work this morning and thought Dr. Blake might enjoy a cookie as well. She apologized for arriving late and explained that her last appointment ran late. She shared that she saw a therapist in her 20s before starting medical school to work through difficulties with her relationship with her mother and sister, but she has been relatively stable throughout residency and fellowship. Katherine acknowledged feeling anxious about seeing a psychiatrist and wasn't sure that she *really* needed to.

A. Salajegheh, MD (✉)
Weill Cornell Medical College/New York-Presbyterian Hospital, New York, NY, USA
e-mail: ans9145@med.cornell.edu

© Springer Nature Switzerland AG 2019   157
J. S. Gordon-Elliott, A. H. Rosen (eds.), *Early Career Physician Mental Health and Wellness*,
https://doi.org/10.1007/978-3-030-10952-3_14

She explained that toward the end of her fellowship, she felt a lump in her breast that was ultimately found to be cancerous. She has since undergone a lumpectomy, chemotherapy, and radiation and is currently taking tamoxifen. She started chemotherapy toward the end of her fellowship and took off 6 months to finish treatment before returning to work a year and a half ago.

Since returning to work as an attending, she finds herself struggling to connect with patients, especially those who "are better off than me." When asked to explain this further, Katherine revealed that she often compares her own illness and prognosis with her patients and finds herself having difficulty locating her empathy when she feels that her patients are "better off" than herself from the perspective of health. She sees patients in outpatient treatment from a variety of backgrounds and with a variety of illnesses, but she has struggled the most with patients who have or have had a history of cancer.

Furthermore, she both worried that her patients can "tell" that she has had a serious illness, and, at other times, she wishes she could tell them about her own experiences. She was concerned that she lost her ability to know how to "be in charge" of a clinical situation. She believes this has caused her to doubt her diagnoses, medication choices, and treatment decisions for her patients.

Finally, she felt certain that she was given her job out of pity. The institution where she trained through residency and fellowship (and is now hired as an attending) felt the need to "take care" of her and would not have hired her on her own merit. She worries that her superiors will realize their mistake and that she will lose her job.

During this session, Dr. Blake asks about Katherine's energy and concentration, and Katherine admitted to having difficulty with both. She added that she has been easily annoyed and often infuriated "when I'm asked to do what is supposed to be my job!" She explained that when asked to complete tasks that are routine, she often finds herself fuming. She has had difficulty falling asleep at night and often bursts into tears, usually of frustration, at seemingly minor irritations (such as locking herself out of her office by accident). She worries about recurrence in the near or distant future, "chemo brain," how she will navigate romantic relationships, issues around fertility, and about student loans and finances.

Throughout her description, Katherine frequently teared up and asked if she can use a tissue from the box on the side table next to her. During the evaluation, Dr. Blake sneezed at one point, and Katherine offered her a tissue.

Principles of Diagnosis and Treatment

Diagnosis

Dr. Blake diagnoses Katherine with generalized anxiety disorder (GAD). Katherine met criteria for this diagnosis as she described excessive and difficult to control worry for at least the past 6 months (and likely longer) affecting her work. Additionally, she described feeling irritable, being easily fatigued, and difficulty falling asleep. She describes difficulty focusing on what her patients are saying in session at times and attempts to compensate for this by drinking multiple cups of coffee per day. She denied having panic attacks, although she does describe a recent episode when, after finally catching a taxi when running late for a dinner, she was overwhelmed with sense of doom, intense nausea (asking the cabdriver to pull over while she dry heaved), shortness of breath, and diaphoresis. This was not in keeping with hot flashes which she has had intermittently since starting tamoxifen.

Katherine's diagnosis is complicated by the fact that she takes tamoxifen daily, and some of the symptoms she describes could be medication side effects. However, Katherine's history reveals that the symptoms have been present at other times in her life, in more or less severe forms, and that she had many of the symptoms during her treatment and prior to starting her tamoxifen. Dr. Blake's differential diagnosis includes panic disorder, major depressive disorder, substance-induced anxiety disorder, and alcohol use disorder.

While Katherine described having had one potential panic attack, this has not been with sufficient frequency or regularity to warrant this diagnosis at this time. Katherine reports tearfulness, feelings of guilt about how her recent illness might be affecting her patients, sleep disturbances, low energy, and poor concentration. There is often overlap with anxiety and depression, and Katherine may, in fact, have a mild depression. Another important consideration is Katherine's caffeine intake. Katherine says that she drinks 4–5 cups of coffee/day to keep up her energy/focus. She has trouble "clearing the fog" in her head when she doesn't drink coffee. Caffeine can contribute to anxiety and mimic symptoms of an anxiety disorder. Lastly, Katherine revealed that she had 3–5 drinks most nights of the week. This had begun during residency and fellowship as most social occasions/ dates revolved around drinking. During cancer treatment, she stopped drinking because of concern about hepatic toxicity, but she resumed drinking on completion of treatment.

Management and Treatment

Generalized anxiety disorder responds best to a combination of medication and therapy. The combination of cognitive behavioral therapy (CBT) and a serotonin reuptake inhibitor (SRI) is most effective in the management of this illness, but other therapy modalities can also be useful including interpersonal therapy, supportive therapy, psychodynamic therapy, and group therapy. Pharmacologically, selective serotonin reuptake inhibitors (SSRIs) are typically first-line treatment, but serotonin-norepinephrine reuptake inhibitors (SNRIs) are also frequently prescribed. While waiting for SRIs to take effect, which can take 3–6 weeks, many patients respond well to low-dose benzodiazepines to help manage acute symptoms of anxiety and insomnia. In Katherine's case, medication choices were limited because of CYP2D6 interactions with tamoxifen.

Principles for Doctors Treating Doctors

In general, doctors are an anxious and obsessional bunch, psychiatrists in particular [1]. Developmentally, physicians' anxious temperaments often contribute to their academic success, organization, and attention to detail which medicine regularly demands, and as such, their anxiety is adaptive. In this case, Katherine's reticence to treat her anxiety relates to her concern that without her anxiety, she will not be compelled to achieve the level of excellence in patient care; she worries she will no longer "go the extra mile." This demonstrates, in Katherine, a meta-anxiety, an attachment to the anxiety such that without it, she imagines she would fail. In fact, she had succeeded with her anxiety intact, but it was the diagnosis of cancer which created a tipping point at which the anxiety was no longer adaptive. It was in exploring her attachment to her anxiety with her provider and her feeling of "giving up" and "surrender" in deciding to take medication she ultimately became comfortable with taking medication to address her anxiety.

Despite having been forced into the patient role with her diagnosis of cancer, Katherine was able to grapple with being a cancer patient in an oncology clinic setting with more ease than with being a psychiatric patient. Receiving treatment outside of her field of expertise, she accepted that she had no choice but to relinquish control of her care. Nonetheless, she still discussed the discomfort of being "manhandled" by physicians who could have been her own classmates. She also expressed concern that the medical advice she was receiving was not based on the latest research and spent a significant amount of time on PubMed researching the answers to her questions and double checking the work of her doctors. She talked about feeling enraged when her primary care doctor was not familiar with the latest research and when her oncologist was not familiar with her case. She feels that she was subject to greater anxiety as a physician patient because she was aware of "all of the things that could go wrong, all of the side effects, all of the risks."

As a psychiatrist treating a patient like Katherine, at times, Dr. Blake often found herself feeling inadequate in her own medical knowledge. It was essential to manage her own feelings of countertransference, recognizing that Katherine's was projecting her own feelings of inadequacy.

Initially in treatment, Katherine struggled more with the diagnosis and the treatment of her anxiety disorder than she said that with her cancer. With cancer, she didn't feel she had a choice about treatment, but with her anxiety, she felt that she was deciding to seek treatment. Dr. Blake explored the concept of choice with Katherine, which ultimately led to her accepting that she was taking her tamoxifen because of her own wishes rather than because it was prescribed and required by her oncologist.

Katherine later revealed to Dr. Baker that she views her cancer diagnosis and subsequent need for treatment as a failure. She thought her body failed to respond to attempts to control its biology and a failure of her work ethic in that she took time off. She admits over time that despite the "hypochondria of medical school," during which time she and her classmates became worried that they had various illnesses as they learned about them, she believed that she was immune to illness. She talked about how, as a doctor, viewed by some patients as being in a position of power, she began to believe the "myth" and found it difficult to believe that she was diagnosed with cancer. She said that it wasn't until she saw the MRI image of her own cancer that she fully believed it was real.

With ongoing supportive and insight-oriented work with Dr. Baker, Katherine was able to explore how her cancer diagnosis was a "wake up call" in her life. She says that up until the point when she was diagnosed, she had pursued her career doggedly, and, as a result, her personal life suffered.

She focused on her decision to give up a chance at a romantic relationship and marriage in her late 20s in order to pursue residency at a competitive program. She expressed grief at what she felt she sacrificed to pursue her career; over time and over many sessions, she began to express curiosity about whether dogged pursuit of her career was in fact a way of avoiding parts of her life which made her uncomfortable.

Katherine's ambivalence about being a psychiatric patient was evident in her lateness to the first session, the gift, and the offering of the tissue. This type of behavior continues in further sessions, where Dr. Blake found that Katherine often evoked a need to care for her doctor. The caretaking behavior is, in turn, counterbalanced with persistent tardiness to appointments. Attempts to discuss this with Katherine were met with great anxiety initially, but she is ultimately able to recognize and identify how her own discomfort with the patient role affected her behavior. This was ultimately useful in her work as a psychiatrist where she met her own patients' resistance with increased empathy and understanding.

Outcome

Katherine began seeing Dr. Blake once a week for supportive therapy. She adapted to the role of psychiatric patient very slowly. Initially, her treatment focused on discussions about her patients and challenges she faced in caring for them. After some time, she was able to focus more on her own inner life and worries about her health in the context of trying to return to "normal life." Long-standing family dynamics which contributed to Katherine's anxiety over many years were explored. She gained some understanding of her need to care for others and be in control of situations and how this informed her decision to be a doctor.

After several sessions and much discussion, she ultimately agreed to take an SSRI and started taking escitalopram, which was titrated to 10 mg with good effect. She also took clonazepam 0.5 mg at bedtime to help quiet her mind and help her fall asleep, but as the SSRI took effect, she eventually used the clonazepam rarely (i.e., prior to a screening mammogram). Katherine talked about feeling torn about how much she struggled taking the very medications she recommended to her patients on a regular basis. Finally, Katherine revealed a pattern of excessive alcohol use (3–5 drinks most nights of the week) which diminished as the treatment progressed. She was able to identify and acknowledge that she used alcohol to treat her symptoms of anxiety.

Pearls
- The patient role—as a medical or psychiatric patient—can be particularly unsettling for physicians.
- All patients including doctors are not immune to concerns and reticence about accepting a psychiatric diagnosis and subsequently starting medication and therapy.
- Self-care is critical to care for others.
- Pay close attention to behavior around the structure of the therapy (tardiness, gifts, comments on appearance, etc.) as these are often clues to the patient's feelings about the treatment and important tools to deepen the treatment.
- Screen for addiction, especially with alcohol, in a nonjudgmental manner. Doctors tend to minimize alcohol use and are highly sensitive to judgment about the use of alcohol or other substances, often worrying about its effect on their careers.

Reference

1. Huang CLC, et al. Risks of treated insomnia, anxiety, and depression in health care-seeking physicians: a nationwide population-based study. Ed. Jain Gaurav. Medicine. 2015;94(35):e1323. PMC. Web. 1 Feb. 2018.

Suggested Reading

Lee YS et al. Cancer incidence in physicians: a Taiwan national population-based cohort study. Ed. Patrick Wall. Medicine. 2015;94(47):e2079. PMC. Web. 1 Feb. 2018.

White A, Shiralkar P, Hassan T, et al. Barriers to mental healthcare for psychiatrists. Psychiatr Bull. 2006;374:1714–21.

Chapter 15
The Case of Simona Moya: Patient Death and Support for the Doctor

Jess Zonana

Case

It is Simona's last week of her inpatient rotation during her second year of psychiatry residency. Her confidence over the course of the year has increased, and most recently, she worked with Dr. Keith Brota, a resident favorite, who has valued her input and dedication to their patients. She has felt more run down in the past few weeks as she prepares for her transition to the third year of residency. She has the usual stressors of wrapping up to leave an inpatient unit while also feeling frustrated by the extra time demands required to get handoff from third-year residents about her outpatient caseload.

Simona gets a page from her attending asking her to go to his office just at the moment she thought she could grab lunch. Dr. Brota is looking serious and sympathetic, so she braces for bad news as she sits down.

J. Zonana, MD (✉)
Weill Cornell Medical College/New York-Presbyterian Hospital, New York, NY, USA
e-mail: jez9004@med.cornell.edu

© Springer Nature Switzerland AG 2019   167
J. S. Gordon-Elliott, A. H. Rosen (eds.), *Early Career Physician Mental Health and Wellness*,
https://doi.org/10.1007/978-3-030-10952-3_15

"I just got news that Grace jumped from her balcony last night, and she died. She went to her first outpatient appointment last week as planned, and then killed herself last night."

Simona feels her eyes start to tear up. "What? What happened?" *How could she?* Simona thinks. *We worked so hard together and she was making plans to go back to school…Oh god, her mother, don't think about her mother.* She really doesn't want to cry in front of an attending, but she is not sure she can prevent it. *Why is Dr. Brota so calm? What's wrong with him? How does he seem so steady all the time?*

She asks a couple of questions to keep him talking, while she tries to keep it together, but his long pauses and searching looks are brutal. She struggles to stay engaged and present without crying. *Get me out of this office.*

Keith Brota, former chief resident and now junior attending and assistant training director, had heard great things about Simona before she joined his service, and he could see what other supervisors had found so special about her. She was funny and engaged, warm but had a dry sense of humor, and picked up on subtleties in patient dynamics that are difficult to teach. Her name had come up at a residency meeting earlier in the year, when the residency director noted that she was a star and hadn't seemed to miss a beat even after she broke her wrist in a car accident last summer.

But on Dr. Brota's service, he had begun to worry that Simona was too easily demoralized by common obstacles in the hospital system. She revealed a more irritable edge when asked to complete a treatment plan or call a consult, and she began to be short with some of the nursing staff, which had never been characteristic of her, at least from what he had heard. So, when he got the news about Grace, in addition to the shock, grief, and anger he was feeling about her death, he also felt concerned how Simona would receive and process this tragedy. The initial meeting was tough, but Keith didn't feel surprised she wanted to keep it short. He avoided classic "debriefing" approaches but encouraged her to reach out to him or others if needed. He spoke with the training director and chief resident, to have them help keep an eye on how she was doing.

Two weeks later, Keith emails Simona to see how she is doing. After two days, she writes back, "Thank you for the email. I have been trying not to let it 'get to me' too much, but it's really impossible. It's so upsetting, but I am not sure talking about it more right now will help. I'm just overwhelmed with starting my work in the outpatient department." Keith pushes for them to meet anyway, and so she offers him a time that week she *believes* is not yet scheduled.

At the meeting, Dr. Brota reviews common reactions to patient suicide and shares some of his own feelings about Grace's death in particular. He asks Simona how she is doing, how she is feeling about work, and whom she has spoken to about the suicide. Simona shares that while she is fulfilling her work obligations and concentrating fine, she feels she is dragging herself to work, feeling disillusioned by the ability of psychiatrists to help anyone, and having some trouble going to sleep at night, often because she replays her last interaction with Grace. Talking to others hasn't really helped anything.

Dr. Brota decides to discuss features of depression, grief, and post-traumatic stress disorder. He also asks if she is experiencing any of these – including suicidal thinking. She dismisses any thoughts of suicide "especially after being on the other end of it," and she denies any changes in appetite, though she is more tired than usual, maybe a little "on edge." She volunteers that she isn't sad or anhedonic, just "disillusioned" or "frustrated." She is going out more with her friends from college which helps distract her, and they like to go to bars, so she has been going out more than usual. She quickly interjects, "But I am never drinking during the day or on my own, so don't worry Dr. Brota." She does worry if she is going to be able to "make it" through third year, but "worrying is nothing new for me."

Principles of Diagnosis and Management

Diagnosis

Patient tragedy can elicit strong emotional responses in trainees and have an impact on their management of other patients, attitudes toward colleagues, and feelings about join-ing their medical specialty. Patient suicide can evoke unique feelings, though medical deaths are no less painful. Resident response to patient deaths can also be a factor in provoking or exacerbating psychiatric illness. Students and residents must manage grief and trauma in their training environment, a unique situation which blurs lines among professional train-ing, need for psychosocial supports, and possible need for psychiatric care.

The supervisory role in residency training demands some ability to assess mental health and mental illness in trainees while also demanding boundaries between roles of supervi-sor and therapist. This case highlights some of the challenges for attending doctors in fulfilling this supervisory role and the need for training programs to provide a structure for emo-tional support and psychiatric referral for residents after patient tragedy.

Dr. Brota's role is supervisory and not as a treating psy-chiatrist, so he recognizes limitations in his capacity to fully assess Simona. With the abridged information, the differen-tial diagnosis must remain broad, and a low threshold for referral is important. Dr. Brota considers the following diag-noses: adjustment disorder, major depressive disorder, acute stress disorder, post-traumatic stress disorder (PTSD), gener-alized anxiety disorder, and alcohol use disorder.

Simona is likely experiencing an adjustment disorder with depressed mood, but she is at risk for a major depressive epi-sode and possibly PTSD. From the information available through Dr. Brota's encounter, she does not yet meet full criteria for a major depressive episode, but her coping strate-gies seem to be falling short, and she is beginning to experi-ence deleterious effects of sleep impairment and fatigue.

It can be challenging to differentiate between a major depressive episode and an adjustment disorder, especially with limited information. Diagnosis of an adjustment disor-der requires that emotional or behavioral symptoms develop in response to an identifiable stressor and that there is either marked distress that is "out of proportion" to the severity of the stressor or there is significant impairment in functioning.

"Normal bereavement" is excluded under this diagnosis. The symptoms also should not be an exacerbation of a pre-existing disorder.

Diagnosis of major depressive disorder requires major symptoms to be present *nearly every day* and for *most of the day* and generally manifests both psychological and physiologic effects. Adjustment disorders classically have less "neurovegetative" manifestations – changes in appetite, sleep, and energy – but the difference can be one of severity and pervasiveness. Both diagnoses require impairment, but for people capable of functioning at a very high level, this can be challenging to detect, and the threshold for concern may need to be lowered to "significant change."

Dr. Brota also felt concerned by the differences between his own observations of Simona and previous reports by his colleagues. She remained an impressive resident, but she seemed to be on a negative trajectory. Her work ethic never wavered, but she was more irritable than others described her. He wondered if she was more affected by the car accident than she initially let on or if other things were going on in her personal life. It was difficult for him to adequately assess her for acute stress disorder or PTSD, but her recent car accident, irritability, change in drinking habits, and the recent news of Grace's violent death caused him to consider this as a real possibility.

Any death can have a huge impact on a resident even if they do not meet criteria for a major psychiatric disorder. Experiencing the death of a child for a pediatric resident or observing multiple trauma patients in an emergency setting or hearing about a violent suicide can trigger stress responses that make a resident more vulnerable to psychiatric symptoms.

Management and Treatment

Simona would benefit from a psychiatric consultation. Without additional information, it is difficult to advise her appropriately on what would be helpful for her to feel better.

While it is reassuring in the immediate sense that she does not report suicidal thinking, psychiatric help should be made available *before* this symptom develops.

Adjustment disorders can respond very robustly to a range of psychotherapies. If there are significant mood or anxiety symptoms that elevate the problem to a major depressive disorder or an anxiety disorder, medications such as serotonin reuptake inhibitors (SRIs) should be considered in addition to psychotherapy. PTSD and alcohol use disorders both have psychotherapeutic and psychopharmacologic therapies that promote recovery.

In addition to the psychiatric referral, other supportive measures can be effective from a training program perspective. Dr. Brota can create or utilize a system of support, formal or informal, to continue to help Simona manage the effects of this tragedy on her professional work. Examples of these support systems and educational curricula are discussed below.

Principles for Doctors Treating Doctors

Patient suicide is a universal fear in the practice of psychiatry and, tragically, a relatively common event. It is painful at any point in one's career, but there are specific vulnerabilities and dynamics that may affect residents and students differently. One meta-analysis reports rates ranging from 31% to 69% of psychiatry residents experiencing a patient suicide [10].

Patient deaths on medical services also have potential for significant negative impact on residents and trainees. More and more medical programs are developing models for addressing loss of patients to support residents to better integrate these experiences in their professional development [2, 6]. Both medical deaths and suicides are potentially high-risk/high-gain moments in the development of physician identities, and it is important to provide supervisory and programmatic support for those students and residents affected.

As a supervisor, Dr. Brota has several important roles in his relationship with Simona. First, he is a supervising attending physician on a clinical service. As assistant training director, he is also a program administrator and mentor to Simona and all the trainees whether they are rotating on his service or not. As part of each of these roles, he holds some obligation to help foster a healthy professional identity in Simona, and this requires attention to Simona's mental health and coping mechanisms.

As the supervising attending on a clinical service, Dr. Brota observed Simona to be a knowledgeable resident, attentive and responsive to patients, and worked with her to develop a wider range of therapeutic approaches. He felt concerned that her occasional irritability in interactions with nursing staff was detrimental to the team culture on the unit and the patient care environment, thus detrimental to her effectiveness. He cautioned her to soften her tone on one or two occasions, which she acknowledged and corrected. She showed up, worked hard, was appropriate with patients, and responded to feedback, so he felt it would be intrusive to push more to address his more subtle concerns with her at the time.

With news of the suicide, Dr. Brota initially met with Simona as he would with any resident – to deliver the news and check in, but not conduct a formal "debriefing" session. During his own training, he had a classmate who had been very angry after a patient suicide, because he felt he had not received the support he needed when family members expressed anger at the treatment team. In response, as chief resident, Dr. Brota organized a program to provide flexible support for residents before and after patient deaths, and this had been well-received in general.

The situation with Simona felt a bit different for Dr. Brota. This was his first patient suicide as an attending, and he was personally shocked by the circumstances of the suicide. The young woman had jumped from her balcony with her mother at home, and while they had discussed suicide risk in depth, the patient had only ever mentioned overdose as a possible method. He was immediately regretful he had not been more forceful in insisting on a more intensive plan for outpatient care. He had recommended such, but the patient was adamant it was more important she go back to school full-time. The patient's mother had acted helpless and passive in the meetings, and she seemed unable or unwilling to ally with him to convince her daughter to participate in a more intensive treatment.

Simona left his service the week following the news of the suicide, and now, a few weeks later, she was already engulfed in her outpatient work. Normally, he would check in with residents a few weeks after a patient suicide, and this time, it felt even more important since he was already worried about her. This was his patient too, after all, and he was still working through his own painful reactions. He kept replaying the family meetings, so they had a different outcome, or rewriting the narrative to keep her in the hospital longer.

Simultaneously, Dr. Brota was also feeling regretful that he hadn't worked harder to engage Simona more meaningfully while she was working with him. She kept a palpable distance and did her work impressively most of the time, so he felt limited in his opportunities to create depth. On the occasions where he could give her feedback in response to a misstep, he did, but these interactions had not led to greater connectivity.

When Dr. Brota sent the follow-up email suggesting they meet, he sensed Simona feeling burdened by his attempts at support. He felt relief when she agreed to meet with him, but he also brought the urgency of his own regret to the meeting. He found it challenging to stay mindful of all the ways his own reactions to the patient suicide and to Simona might be affecting his decisions in how to be helpful to her.

He decided it was important and appropriate to discuss her overall mental health with her, even if she was sending distancing signals. While he realized he might be enacting some corrective impulse from the patient suicide, he also felt it was an important part of his supervisory role to make sure she was getting all forms of support she might need – social, professional, and psychiatric. While it was not his role to provide therapy, it was his role to help her consider that therapy might be beneficial to her at this point.

In hindsight, Dr. Brota wondered if he should have facilitated a meeting for Simona with someone else from the education team. His roles of supervisor and administrator in this case were further complicated by the fact that Dr. Brota shared in the grief over this patient. This potentially offered a means for connection and support between colleagues, but it also made for tricky role straddling and countertransference enactments.

Residency training programs are also charged with multiple responsibilities. They are employers tasked with training competent physicians, but they are also charged with overseeing the development of physician identities in a broad sense. Addressing trainees' personal mental health is impossible to separate out entirely from this process.

More and more, training programs are recognizing the importance of preparing residents for patient deaths and the psychological impact of these tragedies [6, 8, 11]. Best practices around preparing for and responding to patient deaths are still being developed and not necessarily obvious. In psychiatry, several examples of educational curricula have been published with data supporting the practice as well-received by residents [1, 5, 7, 8, 9]. Emerging practices in education include inviting family members of patients who died by suicide to speak to trainees, having psychiatrists share their experiences coping with patient suicide, discussing peer- or incident-review processes, and preparing residents for common emotional reactions.

Less consensus exists on how to provide a programmatic structure for emotional and professional support for residents following specific patient deaths. Medical specialties, such as pediatrics and oncology, are also sharing models for resident support following patient deaths. It is clear that offering support of some kind is important, but there is still cause for concern over the practice of formal "debriefing" after patient tragedy or any potentially traumatic situation. Some programs have published that this practice has been helpful to trainees [2], while other studies have indicated this practice might be potentially harmful to residents – resulting in *increased* symptomatology of acute stress disorder or post-traumatic stress disorder [4].

In both suicide and medical death, most supervisors and programs recommend including residents in any family meetings and family contact following patient death. While there can be no one-model approach, most residents surveyed have found this to be important in the grieving and healing process [3, 5].

Incident review processes and Morbidity and Mortality (M&M) conferences also have the potential to be helpful or harmful. Providing preparation and support for trainees through this process is an important opportunity for support. Members of these committees conducting investigations are not necessarily attuned to the needs of residents, and the way they inquire about the incident may be upsetting to those in conflict after patient death.

Should residency programs be responsible for promoting and supporting the mental health of their residents? Yes. But the answers become more challenging when the questions get more specific – to what extent should programs be actively screening and monitoring the mental health of their residents? This can be intrusive and potentially discriminatory. Having an accessible system to facilitate psychiatric care is important, but how do you normalize it so that residents use it? How do you provide enough coverage, so residents *can* use it?

Accessing and affording mental health care is a challenge for most people, and physician training is in the midst of a culture shift in how to both protect and demand their trainees' time. Having system for psychiatric referrals for residents and trainees is extremely important. These systems are neutralized if residents can't access them because of time demands, stigma, or cost.

Outcome

Dr. Brota recommends to Simona that she meet with a psychiatrist and consider psychotherapy in addition to any other treatments she and doctor might decide are indicated. He shares his perspective that psychotherapy assists in both personal and professional development for residents training to be psychiatrists. He is careful not to diagnose her in this context of supervision, though notes the importance of doctors learning to reflect on their own mental and physical functioning.

Dr. Brota facilitates contact between Simona and the House Staff Mental Health referral system, and she meets with a psychiatrist 2 weeks later. She starts psychotherapy once weekly and then decides with her psychiatrist to start escitalopram several weeks later.

Two months later, Simona sends Dr. Brota an email, letting him know she is feeling much better, thanking him for meeting with her earlier in the year. She states she still gets anxious when meeting with patients who remind her of Grace, but she is feeling more engaged in her work and less burdened by all she must do.

Pearls
- Clinical and academic supervisors can play a role assessing the mental health of their residents.
- Residents experience a supportive training environment when a curriculum is offered to prepare for patient death and suicide and when a program for support is present following patient deaths.
- Harmful vs. helpful elements of formal "debriefing" sessions remain unclear, so caution still advised.
- Supervisors and training programs should have a low threshold for psychotherapy and psychiatry referrals – earlier intervention leads to less impairment and distress.
- Residency training programs should publicize their mental health referral system and create usable clinical coverage plans to allow residents to utilize referrals.

References

1. Cazares PT, Santiago P, Moulton D, Moran S, Tsai A. Suicide response guidelines for residency trainees: a novel postvention response for the care and teaching of psychiatry residents who encounter suicide in their patients. Acad Psychiatry. 2015;39:393–7.
2. Eng J, Schulman E, Jhanwar SM, Shah MK. Patient death debriefing sessions to support residents' emotional reactions to patient deaths. J Grad Med Educ. 2015;7(3):430–6.
3. Granek L, Bartels U, Barrera M, Scheinemann K. Challenges faced by pediatric oncology fellows when patients die during their training. J Oncol Pract. 2015;11(2):e182–9.
4. Hollingsworth C, Wesley C, Huckridge J, Finn G, Griksaitis M. Impact of child death on paediatric trainees. Arch Dis Child. 2018;103:14–8.
5. Jefee-Bahloul H, Hanna RC. Teaching psychiatry residents about suicide loss: impact of an educational program. Acad Psychiatry. 2014;38:768–70.
6. Khot S, Billings M, Owens D, Longstreth WT Jr. Coping with death and dying on a neurology inpatient service: death rounds as an educational initiative for residents. Arch Neurol. 2011;68(11):1395–7.
7. Lerner U, Brooks K, McNiel DE, Cramer RJ, Haller E. Coping with a patient's suicide: a curriculum for psychiatry residency training programs. Acad Psychiatry. 2012;36:29.
8. Mangurian C, Harre E, Reliford A, Booty A, Cournos F. Improving support of residents after a patient suicide: a residency case study. Acad Psychiatry. 2009;33(4):278.
9. Prabhakar D, Balon R, Anzia JM, Gabbard GO, Lomax JW, Bandstra BSY, Eisen J, Figueroa S, Theresa G, Ruble M, Seritan AL, Zisook S. Helping residents cope with patient suicide. Acad Psychiatry. 2014;38:593–7.
10. Puttagunta R, Lomax ME, McGuinness JE, Coverdale J. What is the prevalence of the experience of death of a patient by suicide among medical students and residents? A systematic review. Acad Psychiatry. 2014;38:538–41.
11. Senthil K, Serwint JR, Dawood FS. Patient end-of-life experiences for pediatric trainees: spanning the educational continuum. Clin Pediatr. 2016;55(9):811–8.

Suggested Reading

Gitlin M. A psychiatrist's reaction to a patient suicide. Am J Psychiatry. 1999;156:10.

Sacks M. When patients kill themselves. Ed. Allan Tasman. Am Psychiatr Press Rev Psychiatry. 1989;8:563–579.

Tsai A, Moran S, Shoemaker R, Bradley J. Patient suicides in psychiatric residencies and post-vention responses: a national survey of psychiatry chief residents and program directors. Acad Psychiatry. 2012;36(1):34–8.

Chapter 16
The Case of Leila Moro: Not Just the Blues

Alyson Gorun and Julie Penzner

Case

Leila Moro, a 29-year-old woman in her third year of internal medicine residency, with no prior psychiatric treatment, presented for a psychiatric evaluation at the urging of her husband, also a resident physician following the birth of their first child and Leila's return to work after a 6-week maternity leave. At baseline, Leila described herself as a determined, accomplished person. She was proud that she matched in a rigorous and competitive residency even though it was located hours away from family. She "never thought I'd need help since I'm a doctor" and was accustomed to "not showing any weakness." She "never complained" while pregnant, despite long hours on her feet. However, upon direct questioning, she disclosed feeling more irritable and sad toward the end of her pregnancy.

Leila delivered a full-term, healthy baby, Sol, via an uncomplicated spontaneous vaginal delivery. After Sol's birth, Leila cried more than she remembered crying at any

A. Gorun, MD · J. Penzner, MD (✉)
Weill Cornell Medical College/New York-Presbyterian Hospital, New York, NY, USA
e-mail: aag9014@nyp.org; jup9010@med.cornell.edu

© Springer Nature Switzerland AG 2019   181
J. S. Gordon-Elliott, A. H. Rosen (eds.), *Early Career Physician Mental Health and Wellness*,
https://doi.org/10.1007/978-3-030-10952-3_16

other point in her life. She found it hard to be around Sol. In the hospital, her obstetrician suggested that she had "post-partum blues" and imagined her symptoms would resolve within 2 weeks. Two weeks later, Leila continued to struggle—she couldn't understand that other new parents felt connected to their infants. She spent much of the day crying. Contrary to her feelings of competence at work, she felt unskilled as a mother and found breastfeeding tiresome and frustrating. She had 6 weeks of maternity leave, while her husband had a 2-week leave. She spent much of the last 4 weeks of her leave feeling resentful that her husband was working. She struggled between a wish to return to work, a domain where she felt proficient, and guilt that she wanted to be anywhere other than with her baby. When Leila returned to work after a 6-week leave, Sol was cared for by a combination of daycare and a babysitter. She hoped that with the intensity of residency, she would forget whatever emotional challenges she was experiencing. This, however, was not the case. Leila felt envious of Sol's babysitter, whom she felt was a more capable "mother." At work, when she had time to pump breastmilk, she found pumping in the bathroom humiliating. She regularly cried while pumping as well as during moments between patient care. Paramount to Leila was a sense that she had to "tough it out" among her colleagues though sleep deprivation made concentrating difficult. One of her attendings commented that she regularly looked as though she was crying and was more irritable with colleagues and patients. She suggested she see a mental health professional. Leila perceived this suggestion as confirmation that she was a "failure." During an ER shift, Leila received a call from Sol's daycare that he vomited. Forced to call in a co-resident from jeopardy, she imagined her colleagues were feeling angry and hostile toward her and her decision to become a parent. She felt like a "burden on everyone," unable to do "anything right," and incompetent as a physician, a colleague, a partner, and a mother. Leila rarely attended Sol's pediatric appointments due to her work schedule. Though had she attended one of his appointments, she may have been screened for a postpartum mood episode. Leila struggled to find time to exercise, sleep, or engage in any self-care. Three months postpartum, she was anhedonic, was unable to sleep even once Sol was sleeping, and, on one occasion, had an intrusive image of losing Sol while taking a walk. While she was distressed by this thought, Leila was also scared to see a psychiatrist. She feared that awaiting her was some sort of confirmation that she was unfit to be a mother and physician. Her husband, aware of her insomnia and crying spells, insisted that she meet with a psychiatrist.

When Leila first presented, her psychiatrist, Dr. Haas, unbeknownst to Leila, was also just returning from her maternity leave. She quickly recognized that the symptoms Leila described were neurovegetative symptoms of depression that necessitated treatment. First, she ruled out a psychiatric emergency—Leila recalled the distressing imagine of losing Sol. She felt helpless and scared and confused by this experience. Dr. Haas appreciated that her thoughts were egodystonic and not psychotic. She evaluated Leila for suicidality and Leila reiterated a wish to live. She did not want to hurt herself or her son. As such, Dr. Haas did not believe that there was indication for hospitalization. During Leila's initial evaluation and subsequent sessions, Dr. Haas focused on concrete strategies for Leila regarding time management and negotiating time off all the while normalizing the extraordinary experience of new parenthood. Although Dr. Haas did not typically deliver directive advice to her patients, she felt a problem-solving approach was necessary to deliver some immediate relief for Leila. Dr. Haas recommended weekly supportive psychotherapy in addition to treatment with a serotonin reuptake inhibitor (SRI). They discussed strategies to make time for treatment. In the midst of Leila's evaluation, Dr. Haas reflected on her own experience with parenthood and that her countertransference would be an important tool in Leila's treatment.

Principles of Diagnosis and Management

Diagnosis

Leila Moro was suffering from a major depressive episode with peripartum onset. This is the most frequent type of perinatal mood disorder and has a prevalence of 10–15% [1]. DSM-5 uses the specifier "peripartum onset" which replaced the specifier "postpartum onset" used in DSM-IV-TR [2, 3]. Peripartum is used and not postpartum, given that many depressive episodes, including Leila's, begin during pregnancy [4]. The "peripartum" specifier can be used if onset of mood symptoms occurred during pregnancy or in the 4 weeks following delivery. Many clinicians extend their consideration of "peripartum" to include up to 1 year following birth though there is no consensus on how long the postpartum period should be [5, 6].

"Postpartum blues" is not included in the DSM but is likely what Leila's obstetricians suggested she was feeling following childbirth. It is a mild syndrome occurring within 2 weeks of delivery that includes crying, irritability, insomnia, and anxiety. Presence of postpartum blues is a known risk factor for a postpartum major depressive episode [7]. Leila's diagnosis is more consistent with major depressive episode than "postpartum blues" because her symptoms persisted past 2 weeks postpartum, were severe enough to interfere with functioning and relationships, and extended beyond irritability and anxiety. Phenomenologically, Leila's perinatal depression included classic symptoms of anxiety and agitation, including obsessional thoughts about the newborn [1]. Among the challenging features of this diagnosis is distinguishing difficulty sleeping and low energy due to tending to the needs of an infant versus symptoms caused by a depressive episode. The Edinburgh Postnatal Depression Scale may help with these questions [5].Other pertinent diagnoses to consider in Leila's case were persistent depressive disorder, depressive disorder due to another medical condition, bipolar disorder, psychosis secondary to a depressive episode versus a primary psychotic disorder, or a substance use disorder. Low mood, anhedonia, insomnia, fatigue, inappropriate guilt, and difficulty concentrating are all suggestive of a major depressive disorder. Although postpartum depression may be a manifestation of bipolar depression [8], Leila denied symptoms or history suggestive of hypomania or mania. Ruling out psychosis is particularly important, as postpartum mood episodes with psychotic features carry elevated risk of infanticide and suicide [9]. Substance use occurs during pregnancy and postpartum periods though Leila denied substance use during her evaluation with Dr. Haas [10].

Management and Treatment

Psychotherapeutic goals for peripartum depression include ego-supportive interventions regarding decision-making, i.e., going back to work or extending one's leave, childcare options, decisions around breastfeeding and/or formula feeding, and prioritizing self-care [1, 11]. Cognitive behavior therapy, interpersonal therapy, perinatal dyadic therapy, and mindfulness-based interventions are all evidence-based psychotherapies that are recommended for treating perinatal depression [1, 11].

Treatment of major depression with peripartum onset is similar to treatment of major depression without peripartum onset. SRIs are first-line pharmacological treatment given safety profile and evidence base for efficacy [11]. The decision to use medication should reflect a discussion between the doctor and patient about the severity of symptomatology, prior response to medications, and the benefit of alternative or combined treatment options [1]. Additional considerations include the possible effect of medication on the fetus (if symptoms emerge during pregnancy) as well as on breastfeeding [11]. In the event that a patient presents with symptoms including psychosis, suicidality, or homicidality or if there is any concern that the mother or child is at risk, this is a psychiatric emergency and hospitalization is indicated.

There are only a few mother-infant hospital units in the United States, making separation an upsetting norm, and mindfulness around this issue is an important part of any treatment intervention.

Principles for Doctors Treating Doctors

Medical school and graduate medical education often occurs during the most fertile part of a woman's life. It is estimated that more than 35% of women will become pregnant during their graduate medical education [12]. Since the establishment of the Bell Commission in 1987, more critical thinking has been placed on resident work hours. At present, residents' work hours are limited to 80 hours per week. Decisions regarding parental leave—whether it is maternity leave or paternity leave—are institution and at time department specific and frequently determined in case-by-case decisions [12]. Some departments offer 6 weeks of leave, while others give up to 12 months of leave [12, 13]. Even among programs with more flexible leave policies, the financial toll of medical education debt and the overall length of medical training often preclude residents from taking their preferred amount of leave time [12, 14, 15]. A psychiatrist treating a postpartum resident should familiarize themselves with their patient's institution or department's leave of absence policies and guidelines on parental leave in order to help their patient plan and utilize resources. Such a directive and practical role may be unfamiliar for providers. Depending on the level of functioning of the patient and need for supportive interventions, the treating psychiatrist may have to wait until practical issues are settled before dynamic conflicts can be explored. Difficulties around childcare, for example, can be addressed by inviting their patient to bring their newborn to appointments. This can also help orient the provider to parent-child interactions and attachments. Furthermore, flexibility around patient's availability, making use of telepsychiatry sessions, and an understanding around the availability of childcare are examples of more lenient boundaries that may ensure treatment adherence.

Practically, at the beginning of an evaluation of any resident physician, or anyone for that matter, treatment must be framed as a confidential, protected space in which confidentiality is always honored unless there is a concern that there is a potential risk to the patient or others. The question of fitness to work, which Leila is concerned could come up in her case, is not the decision of one's psychiatrist. Rather, one's ability to work is a decision made by one's residency program leadership in conjunction with an institution's department of occupational health as well as collateral information from one's treating psychiatrist. This highlights the tension between confidentiality and graduate medical education policies with the goal of ensuring that resident physicians receive the care and support they need in order to safely function as a physician.

Pregnancy and parenthood are unique medical and life events. Pregnant residents as well as residents deciding to become parents during residency via surrogacy or adoption often perceive their decision to have a child during residency as one that is burdensome toward colleagues. Namely, the new parent must prepare others for their leave and this can often perpetuate additional guilt [14]. For some, this may manifest with avoidance around feelings of vulnerability and dependency and prompt one to take on increased responsibility following return from maternity leave [16, 17]. Feelings of lack of control at home and at work (i.e., one's call schedule, an infant's sleep patterns) can feel particularly overwhelming to an expecting or new parent. This may be mitigated by increasing control in other areas such as by completing requirements early or doing a year of research between clinical years. Providers should become familiar with resources that can be accessed from home including online support groups (e.g., Postpartum Support International) and CBT workbooks such as *The Pregnancy and Postpartum Anxiety Workbook* [18].

A review paper by Finch outlines challenges specific to pregnant and postpartum residents, including unpredictable schedules, long work hours, lengthy in-house call, fatigue, and sleep deprivation [19]. In addition, issues related to childcare, developing outside support networks and managing breastfeeding and/or pumping, are additional stresses that may impact one's psychological well-being [14]. Residents' schedules afford limited accommodation for the demands of parenthood. The treating doctor should be aware, however, that the patient's difficulty engaging in care may also be a manifestation of conflicts around assertion, self-care, boundary setting, and dependency. Difficulty with scheduling psychiatric appointments can be managed creatively, including using post-call time, conference time, or lunch for appointments. If a resident continues to struggle with scheduling, it is important for the psychiatrist to tend to underlying conflicts impacting a patient's engagement in treatment. This may be related to the transition from caretaker to patient as well as the transition from resident to resident and parent.

A physician, for example, whose identity was largely informed by the hard work and hours dedicated to work in the hospital, may feel guilty enjoying a new role at home with a child. Alternatively, one may feel that their desire to work instead of spending time at home makes one an unsuited parent [17]. Efforts to subvert one's conflict between work and home become particularly difficult given the physical and emotional demands of parenthood. Subtle and overt messages shaming parents at work, including but not limited to ostracizing one for talking about one's children during the work day, inadequate breastfeeding or pumping facilities, and limited daycare options, all impact the experience of returning to work following parental leave [14].

Young and typically healthy physicians are unaccustomed to the patient role which can generate resistance to medication and/or therapy. In turn, conflicts related to dependency may be experienced as humiliating. Reliance on external supports, including a spouse, babysitter, daycare, family, colleagues, and psychiatrist, may be particularly difficult for obsessional physicians who are frequently trained to assert control and autonomy. Independence and ownership that propelled professional successes can inhibit one's capacity to identify the role for support.

Pregnancy, the postpartum period, and parenthood in young physicians can stir up competition, jealousy, aggression, and envy. One's personal goals can feel pitted against professional ones. Colleagues may imply that a physician on leave has been "on vacation," has less professional focus, and is behaving in a way that is negligent toward their colleagues [16, 17]. Resentment may also manifest in the provider's countertransference. Perhaps the treating psychiatrist had difficulty conceiving, wishes that he or she could extend their parental leave, or feels guilty about the resources and supports that he or she identified that their patient is struggling to access. Alternatively, a psychiatrist may feel competitive with their patient's professional success. Understanding the limitations of external comparisons for self-esteem and identity regulation relieves tension for the provider and improves the treatment [17].

Outcome

Leila's initial treatment focused on several practical issues. Leila, along with Dr. Haas and Sol's pediatrician's support, opted to stop breastfeeding and pumping. She was able to reduce sleep deprivation and conflicts in her schedule. She also negotiated for 1 year of part-time residency. Although her training was extended by a year, her increased time at home was the right choice for her psychological well-being. Notably, the attending who commented on Leila's symptoms shared that she too made a similar decision following her first child's birth. For Leila, she experienced having a professional role model with similar conflicts as giving her "permission" to manage her experience and feel reassured of a successful professional outcome. When Dr. Haas had to cancel a session to tend to her own childcare needs, Leila subsequently canceled multiple sessions. Dr. Haas interpreted her behavior in the context of Leila's difficulty with dependency. Leila gained insight with regard to her own conflicts regarding accepting support and competition with another working mother. As a result, Leila became more adept at managing boundaries at work, internalizing that she was a "good enough" physician and mother, and identifying and advocating for her needs. Leila also benefited from a SRI. With time, Leila appreciated the lifting of her depression and fulfillment from her caretaking responsibilities as a physician and mother.

Pearls
- There are unique stressors to the physician parent that include unpredictable schedules, long work hours, sleep deprivation, strict requirements for training, and financial debt.
- Supportive interventions and concrete suggestions may be necessary at the beginning of treatment in order to ensure adherence.
- Clear delineation of the role as the patient's physician and not as a reporter to residency directors or occupational health.
- Major psychological conflicts for physicians in training who return from paternity leave include professional versus maternal identity, dependency versus caretaking, and inadequacy versus competency.
- Countertransference issues may include competition, aggression, and envy. Using countertransference to understand the patient's experience may be useful therapeutically.

References

1. Meltzer-Brody S, Jones I. Optimizing the treatment of mood disorders in the perinatal period. Dialogues Clin Neurosci. 2015;17(2):207–18.

2. American Psychiatric Association. Diagnostic and statistical manual of mental disorders. VI-TR ed. Washington: American Psychiatric Publishing; 2000.
3. American Psychiatric Association. Diagnostic and statistical manual of mental disorders. 5th ed. Washington: American Psychiatric Publishing; 2013.
4. Yonkers K, Ramin S, Rush A, Navarrete C, Carmody T, March D, Heartwell S, Leveno K. Onset and persistence of postpartum depression in an inner-city maternal health clinic system. Am J Psychiatry. 2001;158(11):1856–63.
5. Committee Opinion No. 630. The American College of Obstetricians and Gynecologists Committee Opinion no. 630. Screening for perinatal depression. Obstet Gynecol. 2015;125(5):1268–71.
6. O'Hara MW, McCabe JE. Postpartum depression: current status and future directions. Annu Rev Clin Psychol. 2013;9:379–407.
7. O'Hara M. Prospective study of postpartum blues. Arch of Gen Psychiatry. 1991;48(9):801.
8. Di Florio A, Forty L, Gordon-Smith K, Heron J, Jones L, Craddock N, Jones I. Perinatal episodes across the mood disorder spectrum. JAMA Psychiatry. 2013;70(2):168.
9. Donahue Jennings K, Ross S, Popper S, Elmore M. Thoughts of harming infants in depressed and nondepressed mothers. J Affect Disord. 1999;54(1–2):21–8.
10. Zuckerman B, Amaro H, Bauchner H, Cabral H. Depressive symptoms during pregnancy: relationship to poor health behaviors. Int J Gynecol Obstet. 1990;31(1):90–1. octors treating Doctors: Wellness in the Formative Years
11. Susser L, Sansone S, Hermann A. Selective serotonin reuptake inhibitors for depression in pregnancy. Am J Obstet Gynecol. 2016;215(6):722–30.
12. Blair J, Mayer A, Caubet S, Norby S, O'Connor M, Hayes S. Pregnancy and parental leave during graduate medical education. Acad Med. 2016;91(7):972–8.
13. Greenfield N. Maternity and medical leave during residency: time to standardize? Int J Womens Dermatol. 2015;1(1):55.
14. Chretien K. Mothers in medicine. 1st ed. Cham: Springer; 2018. p. 21–30.
15. Jagsi R, Tarbell N, Weinstein D. Becoming a doctor, starting a family — leaves of absence from graduate medical education. N Engl J Med. 2007;357(19):1889–91.

16. Auchincloss E. Conflict among psychiatric residents in response to pregnancy. Am J Psychiatry. 1982;139(6):818–21.
17. Tinsley J. Pregnancy of the early-career psychiatrist. Psychiatr Serv. 2000;51(1):105–10.
18. Wiegartz P, Gyoerkoe K. The pregnancy and postpartum anxiety workbook: practical skills to help you overcome anxiety, worry, panic attacks, obsessions, and compulsions. Oakland: New Harbinger Publications; 2009.
19. Finch S. Pregnancy during residency. Acad Med. 2003;78(4):418–28.

Suggested Reading

Butts N, Cavenar J. Colleagues' responses to the pregnant psychiatric resident. Am J Psychiatr. 1979;136(12):1587–9.

Cox J, Holden J, Sagovsky R. Detection of postnatal depression: development of the 10-item Edinburgh Postnatal Depression Scale. Br J Psychiatry. 1987;150:787–6.

Cullen-Drill M. The pregnant therapist. Perspect Psychiatr Care. 2009;30(4):7–13.

National Institute of Child Health. The relation of child care to cognitive and language development. Child Dev. 2000;71(4):960–80.

Postpartum Support - PSI. Home | Postpartum Support - PSI. 2018. [online] Available at: http://www.postpartum.net/. Accessed 25 Feb 2018.

Chapter 17
The Case of Shilpa Shah: The Complexities of Training an Immigrant Physician

Nisha Mehta-Naik

Case

Dr. Payal Patel is a South Asian-American psychiatrist working in the house staff mental health program for a large academic medical center with several community hospital affiliates. Dr. Patel received a call from the house staff mental health director, saying, "I have a new patient I'd like to send your way. I'm hoping you can relate to Shilpa and be the best qualified to help." Without more information, Dr. Patel felt at first taken aback – recognizing the Indian first name, and thinking *does some shared background inherently make me best qualified to work with Shilpa? Can I relate to Shilpa's experience? Though I am South Asian, I was born in America, with a different cultural upbringing. Does relating to a patient always positively impact the treatment?* She listened carefully to the story, as collected by the house staff mental health director.

N. Mehta-Naik, MD (✉)
Weill Cornell Medical College/New York-Presbyterian Hospital, New York, NY, USA
e-mail: nim9063@med.cornell.edu

© Springer Nature Switzerland AG 2019   193
J. S. Gordon-Elliott, A. H. Rosen (eds.), *Early Career Physician Mental Health and Wellness*,
https://doi.org/10.1007/978-3-030-10952-3_17

Dr. Shilpa Shah recently emigrated from Gujarat, India, to pursue a pediatrics residency at an academic community hospital in an urban setting. In her third month of intern year, she was scheduled to see a 6-month-old infant for a routine outpatient clinic visit. In the beginning of the encounter, the baby's mother repeatedly asked Shilpa, "Where are you from? No...where are you *really* from?!" Shilpa recognized that her accent drew attention, and she tried her best to ignore scrutiny surrounding this. When Shilpa inquired about breastfeeding practices, the patient's mother seemed offended by this line of questioning and began to shout. Shilpa was reluctant to ask for help, due to concern that it would reflect poorly on her clinical performance. Within minutes, the mother grabbed her child and charged out of the room, pushing nurses to the side. Nurses approached Shilpa angrily, "Couldn't you tell!? She was drunk! She reeked of alcohol! You should've called us earlier!" Shilpa was stunned – she had never smelled alcohol in her life, nor had she previously needed to manage an episode of agitated behavior.

The charge nurse brought this incident to the attention of the clinic supervisor, who later approached Shilpa. The supervisor expressed concern that the intern not only missed warning signs of escalating agitation but also failed to inform child protective services. When Shilpa attempted to explain that she was not familiar with signs of alcohol intoxication, her supervisor told her, dismissively, that this "was not a good excuse." Her supervisor contacted the residency training program director, expressing concern about Shilpa's patient care deficiencies. After meeting with Shilpa, the program director referred her to the house staff mental health program because Shilpa seemed "anxious and defensive."

At the beginning of their first visit, Shilpa asked Dr. Patel, "Are you from Gujarat? I saw your last name, and it is common where I am from." When Dr. Patel explored her curiosity about a possible shared heritage, Shilpa expressed comfort in meeting someone from India. She also indicated some concern that their families may be social acquaintances in Gujarat and that the details about these recent events might be revealed to them. Dr. Patel explained that the content of their conversation would remain confidential.

Shilpa described feeling misunderstood by her supervisors. "My clinic director didn't even believe me when I told him I did not know about alcohol!" Dr. Patel was surprised that Shilpa missed such blatant signs of intoxication and found herself automatically thinking, too, that shilpa was making "excuses." Dr. Patel gently inquired further, recognizing that though she was Gujarati-American, she was not aware of Gujarat's alcohol policies. Shilpa explained that she was raised in Gujarat, India, a state in which alcohol use and sales remain prohibited. As a result, topics regarding alcohol were not covered in her medical school curriculum, nor did she witness alcohol intoxication in her upbringing.

Dr. Patel opened up the conversation further, asking, "What's it like learning medicine in a whole different culture?" Beginning residency and moving to the United States proved to be more challenging than Shilpa had anticipated. Though she had attended English-medium schools in India and was fluent in the language, she did not yet feel confident conversing in English with native English speakers, including colleagues or patients. She was enjoying the independence of living alone, though often felt lonely and was slowly acclimating to the ins and outs of banking, grocery shopping, and commuting. She often felt like a burden on local family friends who were helping her transition. She recognized that she was progressing slower than her fellow co-interns and felt that her clinical work was being more closely scrutinized.

She admitted that since childhood, a lot of her sense of achievement has come from her performance in school and work. With her recent difficulty transitioning to residency, she reported increased self-critical thinking, ruminative worry, and feelings of worthlessness for the past 3 months. She denied symptoms of panic. She wished she could confide in her family in India, though felt ashamed to inform them of her struggles. She reported sleeping 5 hours nightly in the setting of long work hours, without difficulty falling asleep; she had no changes in concentration, energy, or appetite. She felt motivated to learn and improve her performance, though was unsure how to go about doing so. She was beginning to develop friendships with co-interns and noted that she had enjoyed having dinner with them last week. She still felt happiness on a daily basis, such as the other day when she found a corner grocery in her neighborhood owned by a family from Gujarat, selling some of her favorite food treats. She denied current or past manic or psychotic symptoms or thoughts of self-harm or harming others. She denied any use of alcohol or other substances.

Principles of Diagnosis and Management

Diagnosis

The most likely diagnosis is adjustment disorder with mixed anxiety and depressed mood, given Shilpa's description of ruminative worry, self-critical thinking, feelings of being a burden, and worthlessness in the setting of beginning intern year 3 months ago in a new country [1]. Major depressive disorder should be considered due to the presence of some cognitive features of depression, as well as reduced self-worth. However, she denied pervasively depressed mood or anhedonia, and does not report the neurovegetative symptoms of depression [1]. Generalized anxiety disorder (GAD) should also be considered due to the feature of ruminative worry about job performance, which she described as difficult to control. If these symptoms arose for the first time, as Shilpa reports, only 3 months ago, this would not be fully consistent with a diagnosis of GAD, which is a more chronic disorder requiring at least 6 months duration. Additionally, she does not have associated physical or cognitive symptoms related to anxiety such as edginess or restlessness, excess fatigue, poor concentration, or irritability, all commonly found in a patient with GAD [1].

Dr. Patel should also consider the possibility that Shilpa does not have a psychiatric diagnosis. One could interpret Shilpa's difficulty adjusting to a new role as a physician, while immigrating to a new country, as a socially normative response to a stressful process. Shilpa was misunderstood by her supervisors, who at times did not appreciate the impact of cultural differences on the practice of medicine. Shilpa was quick to recognize that her cultural knowledge deficits were impacting her interactions with patients and her overall residency performance. However, her inability to overcome this deficit within months of immigrating was a tremendous source of stress, and perhaps resulted in her becoming defensive at times Shilpa not only questioned her abilities as a physician, but also carried anxiety about her status in her program and – moreover – in the country, given her current employment-based immigrant visa status. Dr. Patel will want to explore and account for the various psychosocial aspects contributing to her presentation prior to offering a psychiatric diagnosis, particularly in the setting of immigration. If overlooked, the psychiatrist may miss out on valuable opportunities to provide the optimal interventions to help Shilpa survive and even thrive.

Management

Shilpa may benefit from therapy to address low mood and anxiety in the setting of a new stressor. Given that a prominent feature of the current stressor is related to a role transition, interpersonal psychotherapy (IPT) might be particularly well-suited to Shilpa's needs. Supportive psychotherapy, including some cognitive behavioral therapy interventions (such as cognitive reframing), could be useful for offering an encouraging space for Shilpa to process her current difficulties and responses and problem-solve about the particular challenges she is facing.

There are features of depression, without evidence of a clear major depressive episode or a pervasive anxiety syndrome causing significant distress or impairment, and therefore it would be reasonable to delay any decisions for pharmacotherapy at this time. If depressive or anxious features worsened or were further revealed over time, an antidepressant medication, such as a serotonin reuptake inhibitor, could be offered to target depressive and anxious symptoms.

The psychiatrist could consider providing feedback to Shilpa's residency program director about the cultural factors that might be complicating Shilpa's adjustment to residency and her interactions with her colleagues and patients. With Shilpa's consent, this could be done directly between the psychiatrist and the program director or indirectly through a representative from the office of graduate medical education or an ombudsmen role in the hospital or medical center, if one exists. If appropriate, Dr. Patel and Shilpa could even work on having Shilpa practice how to talk to her program director, and perhaps others, about her adjustment in a way that is open, constructive, and receptive to input. To support her transition, the program might assign Shilpa a mentor whose role would be to review cultural issues that emerge in clinical cases, provide education regarding cultural norms, and even guide Shilpa in role playing of interactions with others for practice and for enhancing her confidence.

Principles for Doctors Treating Doctors

Effective training of immigrant physicians is important for assuring the wellness of the medical community, and the health of the American people. More than a quarter of United States physicians were born elsewhere, thus composing a sizeable portion of healthcare providers for the US population [2]. International medical graduate (IMG) physicians are responsible for the healthcare of a large proportion of the US population; in 2005–2006, IMG physicians managed 24.6% of all physician outpatient visits and particularly played an important role in the healthcare of vulnerable groups [3]. When compared to non-IMG physicians, IMG physicians treated a greater percentage of patients from minority backgrounds, as well as those utilizing Medicaid or state children's health insurance programs, and were more likely to practice in geographical regions with shortages of primary care physicians [3].

When evaluating immigrant trainees for mental health issues, psychiatrists should consider psychosocial factors that may contribute to their presentation. Immigrant physicians not only face the challenge of assimilating into the culture of medicine, as do all physicians in early stages of training, but also adjest to a culture of a new country. While Shilpa's case does not represent the experiences of all young immigrant physicians, some challenges are shared. IMG residents acclimate to learning clinical medicine in a foreign country with new curricula, educational styles, and clinical practices. Interviews with IMG physicians highlighted "insensitivity and isolation in the workplace," [4], as well as "themes of struggles for acceptance, fear of rejection, and fear of disappointing patients" [5]. Many immigrant physicians also describe feelings of guilt for leaving, and not serving, their motherland. Additionally, difficulty navigating post-residency career plans in light of visa restrictions further complicates the experience of immigrant physicians.

These unique shared challenges can threaten the healthy educational experience of IMG trainees. Self-motivated and proactive learning, as per adult learning theory, requires an environment that nurtures autonomy, competence, and relatedness [6]. It can initially be difficult for immigrant trainees to feel competent when communicating in a foreign language in which they are not yet fully confident conversing. Moreover, immigrant trainees may not experience a sense of community and relatedness when surrounded by colleagues and patients whose culture is foreign and far removed from a community to which they feel most connected. Autonomy can feel unattainable immediately after entering a new country and new healthcare system, though can be gradually achieved with guidance and education.

An indirect and uncomfortable potential result of efforts paid to enhance these trainees in their transition is the development of resentment among co-residents and supervisors – with immigrant trainees initially perceived as "more work" for the training program and department. Such feelings of resentment may remain unconscious due to their social unacceptability, or be felt but not expressed, and possibly acted out through negative interactions with the trainees or other maladaptive behavior. On the other hand, the addition of members of other cultures can add to the richness of the medical community and its learning and working environment for trainees, faculty, staff, and patients. Creating a network of peer and faculty mentors, providing education specific to American culture and healthcare, while simultaneously offering a sense of community, can help facilitate this process for all involved [4]. A similar model utilizing a network of peer, on-site, and off-site supervisors has been proven to be effective in the career development of underrepresented minorities in medicine [7].

One should also consider psychological factors that may contribute to the immigrant trainee's presentation, some of which are unique to the individual, while some are more clearly influenced by the culture with which one most closely identifies. Shilpa's way of thinking about and engaging in her environment may be impacted by the Hindu concept of *dharma*, which emphasizes the importance of fulfilling one's duty. Shilpa viewed completing medical training in the United States as her "duty" to her family and society. Failure to achieve *dharma* may have contributed to Shilpa's feelings of shame and her reluctance to reach out to her family for support. Culture-independent psychological factors also likely contributed to Shilpa's difficulties. Shilpa described deriving self-esteem from her work performance, and endorsed feelings of worthlessness in the setting of poor performance. She at times had difficulty asking for help when appropriate, as it felt too damaging to her self-image. Such suggestions of instability of self-identity, disruptions in object relations, and need for validation from others, may reflect underlying Kohutian narcissistic traits from a self-psychology perspective [8].

In regard to the psychiatric treatment of immigrant trainees, the treating psychiatrist should consider transference and countertransference reactions which may be impacted by culture and the cultural transition. Factors such as attitudes regarding mental health in the trainee's home country, the trainee's confidence and proficiency in speaking English, and cultural perspectives on hierarchy and authority will shape the immigrant trainee's experience of the encounter with the psychiatrist. Transference responses may include feelings of being scrutinized or judged (which may lead to behavioral reactions such as performing for the psychiatrist or becoming more guarded) or of being in the subordinate position (potentially prompting a sense of being protected and cared for, or of discouragement or constraint). If working with a nonimmigrant psychiatrist, the trainee may have a sense of resentment or envy toward the psychiatrist for not having to face the same life obstacles the trainee has. One may feel misunderstood by the psychiatrist, particularly if the psychiatrist is not mindful of the patient's cultural identity. Other transferences may emerge when the treating psychiatrist belongs to a similar cultural background. Though overidentification is already a common treatment challenge in a doctor-doctor treatment relationship, this may be heightened if the immigrant trainee culturally identifies with their psychiatrist, leading to behaviors that can at times enhance the therapeutic efficacy of the treatment, or impede it.

Certain countertransference responses may emerge as well. Dr. Patel, for example, may feel uncomfortable or aggrieved for being racially profiled by a colleague and labeled as the best suited to treat South Asian patients. This resentment may be unconsciously displaced onto the patient. If from a similar culture background, the psychiatrist may also overidentify with the patient. This may result in the psychiatrist making incorrect assumptions about the patient or normalizing psychological traits and behaviors that could be worthy of clinical attention. When thinking of transference and countertransference reactions, one should keep in mind that both the patient and therapist may have implicit biases about race and skin color, language and accent, and various associations to culture and ethnicity, which could be influenced by cultural values or lifetime experiences. Such biases can impact the psychiatrist's view of the patient and vice versa [9]. The psychiatrist will benefit from continued awareness of, and reflection on, such biases, and how they impact the treatment.

Supervision for the psychiatrist should be encouraged as a way to understand how countertransference responses, biases, and knowledge (or limitations thereof) regarding the immigrant trainee's background are influencing the therapeutic relationship and the treatment response. Feelings of discomfort or anxiety may be present for the psychiatrist who senses being "out of my league" in terms of understanding the cultural factors that are affecting the patient's presentation and the treatment. It may feel uncomfortable or even threatening to seek out a supervisor or a colleague with experience in this area – potentially raising concerns in the psychiatrist about demonstrating clinical insufficiencies or shameful attitudes and prejudices. Such concerns may lead to delay or avoidance of getting help that will benefit both the psychiatrist and the immigrant trainee patient. The psychiatrist can reframe these concerns by approaching the seeking of supervision with an emphasis on openness and curiosity and an expressed eagerness to learn from the colleague or other professional.

Outcome

Shilpa began a course of IPT to address symptoms of low mood and anxiety in the setting of a recent life transition. Shilpa was not initiated on psychiatric medications. Over several weeks, she described feeling more confident, with decreased ruminative worry. She recognized that multiple life events, namely, immigrating and beginning internship, impacted her mood. She was better able to assert herself, felt more comfortable asking questions to co-residents and attendings, and began to develop new networks of social supports while maintaining previous ones. The house staff mental health director reached out to Shilpa's residency program director and suggested that Shilpa be assigned a peer and faculty supervisor to aid her transition to learning medicine in a new country. Shilpa found these supervisors to be educational and supportive. Shilpa's clinical performance gradually improved during her intern year. In her second year of residency, she became a peer supervisor to an intern, who recently immigrated to the United States.

Pearls
- The training of immigrant physicians is not only important in assuring the wellness of the medical community but also the health of the American population.
- When evaluating immigrant trainees, psychiatrists should consider psychosocial factors that may contribute to their presentation, including challenges related to immigration.
- In regard to the psychiatric treatment of immigrant trainees, the treating psychiatrist should consider transference and countertransference reactions which may be impacted by culture.

References

1. American Psychiatric Association. Diagnostic and statistical manual of mental disorders. 5th ed. Arlington: American Psychiatric Publishing; 2013.
2. Castillo-Page L. Diversity in the physician workforce: facts and figures. Association of American Medical Colleges. Supplemental Table 4g. 2010. https://www.aamc.org/download/432976/data/factsandfigures2010.pdf.
3. Hing E, Lin S. Role of international medical graduates providing office-based medical care: United States, 2005–2006. NCHS Data Brief. 2009;13:1–8.

4. Chen PG, Curry LA, Bernheim SM, et al. Professional challenges of non-U.S.-born internal medical graduates and recommendations for supporting during residency training. Acad Med. 2011;86(11):1383–8.
5. Fiscella K, Roman-Diaz M, Lue BH, et al. Being a foreigner, I may be punished if I make a small mistake': assessing transcultural experiences in caring for patients. Fam Pract. 1997;14:112–6.
6. Ryan RM, Deci EL. Intrinsic and extrinsic motivations: classic definitions and new directions. Contemp Educ Psychol. 2000;25:54–67.
7. Lewellen-Williams C, Johnson V, Deloney L, et al. The POD: a new model for mentoring underrepresented minority faculty. Acad Med. 2006;81(3):275–9.
8. Baker M, Baker H. Heinz Kohut's self psychology: an overview. Am J Psychiatr. 1987;144(1):1–9.
9. Tummala-Narra P. Skin color and the therapeutic relationship. Psychoanal Psychol. 2007;24(2):255–70.

Chapter 18
The Case of Edward Thad: An Ethical Dilemma

Charles W. Shaffer and Janna S. Gordon-Elliott

Case

Edward Thad, a 25-year-old MD/PhD student at a highly ranked medical school, was brought by ambulance to the psychiatric emergency department (ED) of the university hospital after sending his advisor provocative text messages referencing suicide. Upon Edward's arrival in the psychiatry ED, a resident standing in the clinician station saw him through the glass screen, recognizing him as a current medical student from a preclinical course the resident had co-facilitated a year prior. The resident alerted Dr. Jensen, the attending that day, who confirmed this information, and then immediately found, and dismissed for the day, the two third year medical students working in the ED as part of their psychiatry rotation. He alerted the dean's office and the director of medical student mental health; and he asked the social worker to arrange for Edward to be assigned an alias in the electronic health record, as per the protocol for student-patients in the psychiatry ED. Dr. Jensen then evaluated Edward on his own without a resident.

C. W. Shaffer, MD · J. S. Gordon-Elliott, MD (✉)
Weill Cornell Medical College/New York-Presbyterian Hospital, New York, NY, USA
e-mail: cws7004@nyp.org; jsg2005@med.cornell.edu

© Springer Nature Switzerland AG 2019
J. S. Gordon-Elliott, A. H. Rosen (eds.), *Early Career Physician Mental Health and Wellness*,
https://doi.org/10.1007/978-3-030-10952-3_18

205

On initial interview, Edward was irritable but in behavioral control. He was alert and appeared physically well. He refused to answer any questions, saying he needed to speak with his advisor first. Dr. Jensen attempted to engage Edward, but his early efforts to build a rapport and gather a history were unsuccessful. When Dr. Jensen returned to the nursing station, he discovered that Edward's advisor had just telephoned, leaving a message that asked for "the senior attending" to call him back as soon as possible.

Collateral was obtained from his advisor, Professor Wilson, and a history emerged. Edward was in his third year of medical school, a year when MD/PhD students move their focus to lab work. Edward had been a somewhat polarizing figure at the medical school dating back to the admission process, during which time questions arose around his inadequately explained undergraduate transfer at the start of his senior year, and the report that a well-liked current MD/PhD student had been "put off" by Edward during a recruitment-related social activity, though the student had chosen not to further explain. With his impressive research background as an undergraduate, superlative letters of recommendations, and strong performance during his interview, the admissions committee accepted him into the program. He had done well academically during the first 2 years of medical school but did not have many close relationships with his classmates.

He began working in Professor Wilson's immunology lab full time 6 months ago. Initially, he impressed everyone as very bright, if somewhat aloof. However, as time went on, Edward fell into conflicts with several other junior researchers in the lab. During lab meetings, he would criticize their work and emphasize the superior approach he was taking. When speaking with Professor Wilson, Edward would complain about not having sufficient access to specialty equipment because it had to be shared with others. Some of these other lab members had reported that Edward was diverting lab supplies allocated to them. Edward's behavior was initially ignored or brushed aside by Professor Wilson, in part because of Edward's apparent talent. Professor Wilson explained to

Dr. Jensen on the phone: "You know, I figured he probably hadn't really figured out how to interact with people that well – that sometimes needs to be part of the training for these students in the lab."

Professor Wilson went on to say that things had changed significantly 1 week prior to Edward's presentation to the ED. There had been a lab-wide meeting during which Edward presented an update on his ongoing work. At the end of the presentation, one of the other lab members and MD/PhD students, Anne, pointed out a significant inconsistency in Edward's early results. Initially, Edward had become irritable and defensive, but when Dr. Wilson interjected to support Anne' criticism, Edward did not argue back, and the meeting ended in an anticlimactic fashion.

Later that evening, Edward sent off dozens of aggressive and vulgar text messages to Anne, disparaging her work and her physical appearance, which she brought to the attention of Professor Wilson the next morning. The night before, Professor Wilson – disturbed by what had occurred during the lab presentation – had spent some time reviewing Edward's notes and raw data, and he was now quite convinced that Edward had been manipulating his results. Not knowing what to do, he decided to tell Edward that he had heard about the texts to Anne and that these were considered unacceptable behavior. He told Edward to "take a few days off," while Professor Wilson discussed the issue with the dean's office; he did not mention that he would also be reviewing the concerns for data manipulation. Edward said little during this conversation and quickly left the office as soon as it was over.

Over the next few days, further information came to light of erroneous data in a manuscript that Edward had been helping one of the lab's postdoctural fellows prepare for publication. The postdoc reported that these data had been Edward's contribution. Professor Wilson and the dean discussed both the unethical misrepresentation of data and the assaultive communication toward a co-student, which was then brought to the attention of the medical school disciplinary committee.

Unaware of much of this, Edward began reaching out to Professor Wilson to state his intention to return to the lab. Initially, Edward acted like nothing had happened and sent a text to Professor Wilson about plans for the next stage of his research project. When Professor Wilson did not reply after a few additional attempts, the tone of Edward's messages changed, becoming more defensive and accusatory. Edward suggested that there had been improprieties in the lab and provocatively mentioned that he was considering "reaching out to" the institutional review board of the medical college.

The next day, after continued silence from Professor Wilson, Edward sent a message that seemed to be a suicide note. At this point, Professor Wilson felt compelled to respond, but when he did not receive a message back, he called 911 requesting a wellness check. When emergency services arrived at Edward's student apartment, he let them in after a brief delay. Prominently visible outside of his bathroom door was a rope that had been loosely tied into a noose-like shape. Edward offered no explanation when asked about the rope, and it was decided to bring him into the ED for further evaluation.

While speaking with Dr. Jensen on the phone, Professor Wilson inquired as to whether he should come to the ED to see Edward. Given Edward's apparent tendency to manipulate and push the boundaries of the relationship, it was recommended that Professor Wilson avoid contact for the time being. After finishing his conversation with Professor Wilson, Dr. Jensen returned to speak with Edward, who had asked the nurse several times when the doctor would be coming back.

Edward was now prepared to talk. He gave a history vaguely similar to that provided by Professor Wilson but with prominent minimizations and omissions. He admitted to having "an anger problem" and acknowledged sending text messages to Professor Wilson and to Anne but stated they had been "taken out of context" and "misinterpreted." He initially denied suicidal ideation but was evasive and provocative when asked about the rope in his apartment, stating that he "just wanted to have options." During the interview, he exhibited an indignant and devaluing attitude. He denied symptoms of depression, and his affect was angry rather than dysphoric. He further denied current or prior symptoms of mania, psychosis, or any history of substance abuse. He was not pressured or disorganized. He denied and did not exhibit any evidence of delusional thinking or perceptual distur-bances. He denied any significant past psychiatric or medical history and took no medications. Routine labs including urine toxicology were within normal limits.

Principles of Diagnosis and Management

Diagnosis

The most appropriate diagnosis in this case is narcissistic per-sonality disorder (NPD). NPD is characterized by "a perva-sive pattern of grandiosity (in fantasy or behavior), need for admiration, and lack of empathy." The DSM-5 diagnostic criteria emphasize aggressive and exploitative externalizing behaviors that may only capture a subset of individuals with NPD. An alternative model proposed in Section 3 of the DSM-5 highlights the psychological structure of the disorder including the characteristically impaired sense of self [1].

In Edward's case, evidence suggests that he demonstrates significant grandiosity and entitlement across multiple set-tings and relationships. This is exemplified by his tendency to devalue the contributions of other colleagues in the lab, as well as his initial idealizing attitude toward Professor Wilson. The subsequent fluctuation in the way Edward relates to his mentor reflects his susceptibility to narcissistic injury and rage, which are hallmarks of the disorder. The core features of NPD, including the need to be seen by others as important, intense underlying insecurity, and deficient capacity for empathy, can lead to inappropriate behavior that may defy social or ethical expectations. Edward's manipulation of data may be understood as an act done to manage his fragile sense of self-esteem, after identifying errors in his work and becoming acutely concerned for being found out for his "failures." While history so far is limited, and more would need to be gathered, there is suspicion that recent events may be part of a pattern of behaviors. For example, his late transfer in college was later identified to be a "face-saving" effort following a never-proven investigation about his having plagiarized an essay. His moments of negative personal interactions with peers, rather than authorities, such as in the social gathering during recruitment, could further support a diagnosis of NPD. His dramatic decompensation leading to his being brought to the ED can be viewed as the consequence of a rare public criticism, which was experienced particularly powerfully since it came from an underestimated colleague and illuminated Edward's shameful dishonesty.

While Edward demonstrates the characteristics of NPD, other diagnoses should be considered. These include bipolar disorder, borderline personality disorder, antisocial personality disorder, and a substance-induced behavioral disorder (such as substance-induced bipolar disorder). His seemingly "abrupt" change in interpersonal behavior, and the poor judgment related to his manipulation of data, could be related to an emerging manic episode. The absence of a psychiatric history would not rule this out, with Edward at an age when bipolar disorder might have its onset (or when an individual who has had depressive episodes may have a first manic episode). He is denying clear manic symptoms, and his exam is not meaningfully consistent with mania, making bipolar disorder a less likely diagnosis. Substance use leading to erratic behavior, either due to repeated intoxication or withdrawal, must be considered; further information could be gathered about his substance use patterns. A negative urine toxicology would lean against this diagnosis, though may not detect substances that have already been eliminated or that are not detected by the screen assay. Compared to borderline personality disorder, NPD is more appropriate since Edward's relationships are mostly characterized by aloof contempt rather than intense dependency or rejection. While Edward demonstrates clear antisocial behavior, the clinical assessment suggests that the psychological need to protect his self-esteem and self-worth is the primary motivator of his behavior, which would be most consistent with NPD, whereas in antisocial personality disorder, the driving force behind antisocial activities is more closely related to their obvious purpose – e.g., stealing property for financial gain or feigning a medical condition to obtain medications that can be sold.

Management

Narcissistic personality disorder is difficult to treat. There is a limited role for medication, but psychotherapy may offer some benefit. Supportive psychotherapy provides a practical, stabilizing approach that works within the bounds of the underlying pathology to optimize resilience, elevate functioning, and guide patients through crises. The advantages of supportive therapy include its wide availability, flexibility, and incorporation of a positive therapeutic relationship that can serve as a model to build interpersonal trust and pro-social behaviors.

In addition, several manual-based therapies have been developed and applied to patients with NPD. The most notable of these include transference-focused psychotherapy (TFP) and schema-focused therapy (SFT). Based on object relations theory, TFP utilizes a psychoanalytically informed approach that strives to bring the patient's psychic structure into consciousness. This is achieved by highlighting the elements of the patient's inner mind as they are "acted out" in the patient's interactions with the therapist. SFT similarly draws on psychodynamic principles, but its roots are in the cognitive behavioral model. Schemas are pervasive unconscious cognitive structures that provide a way to understand and experience oneself and the environment. Schema theory describes personality disorders, including NPD, in terms of early maladaptive schema which are derived from childhood experiences but continue to frame an individual's perception of the world throughout life. SFT is directive and supportive, employing a number of techniques including "limited reparenting" to uncover and provide a more adaptive set of schemas. Both TFP and SFT are long-term therapies that offer the promise fundamental change in the patient's personality structure. While they have been primarily studied in the treatment of borderline personality disorder, there is some evidence that they are effective in NPD, too [2, 3].

Careful assessment for the presence of co-occurring psychiatric disorders is essential for effective management. Commonly, a co-occurring condition, such as depression or a substance use disorder, will be more acutely amenable to treatment, allowing for careful assessment of the personality traits with improvement of confounding disorders, followed by engagement in more long-term treatment to address the personality disorder. Notably, NPD has a strong association with completed suicide, and the risk is increased after negative life events [4, 5], making ongoing safety assessments and safety planning a vital aspect of the treatment plan, both short and long term.

There are no clinical trials on psychopharmacological treatment of NPD. In the absence of co-occurring mood disorders, medications are generally not recommended. Some psychiatrists will use mood stabilizers or atypical antipsychotics for severely dysregulated or aggressive patients. The rationale for these agents is based on clinical experience and data from studies on related cluster b personality disorders (e.g., borderline personality disorder).

Principles for Doctors Treating Doctors

This is an instance of unethical behavior, which – brought to attention – requires an action plan which may include many facets, including investigating the extent and significance of the behavior/breach, following appropriate policy regarding this investigation, identifying the problems in the system and individuals involved, and disciplining the perpetrators. Where relevant, it is also important to identify any confounding factors that may have contributed to the perpetrator's behavior, such as a psychiatric condition. In this case, behavior escalated to the extent that the perpetrator was brought to psychiatric attention. In other cases, the administration and educational leadership may want to consider whether the perpetrator should be encouraged, or required, to have further psychiatric assessment.

In addition to NPD, diagnoses that may be associated with unethical transgressions include antisocial personality disorder, substance use disorder, and bipolar disorder. It is important to identify psychiatric disorders in such cases since treatment may improve outcomes of clinical significance. In certain circumstances, the presence of a psychiatric disorder may also be a mitigating factor when considering disciplinary responses to ethical violations. This is particularly true for first time offenses and less egregious behavior that occurred before the disorder was diagnosed. The question of whether treatment is likely to prevent subsequent incidents is also relevant, as is the availability, practicality, and the individual's acceptance of such treatment. For example, bipolar disorder is defined by episodic deviations from baseline functioning and frequently responds very well to medications. On the other hand, the antisocial behavior associated with personality disorders inherently reflects a maladaptive baseline that is challenging to treat.

In Edward's case, NPD contributed to the ethical violation. While one might assume that NPD would be rare among medical students and physicians, that is not necessarily the case. Entry to medical school (particularly to a research program) requires a degree of accomplishment, assertiveness, and self-confidence that is also seen in NPD. Individuals with NPD can often make a positive first impression, and they may perform particularly well in interviews, where their tendency to "sell themselves" is an advantage. The idealizing attitude that narcissists often show toward people with impressive accomplishments and credentials can also work to their advantage. Mentors may find this flattery alluring and look favorably on them, at least initially.

At the same time, individuals with NPD are not able to "conceal" their personality traits over the course of multiple interactions. Indeed, the diagnosis implies deficient insight, and so the individual may not realize there is anything necessary to conceal. In Edward's case, there are several early clues that distinguish him from most other students that may raise concern. The fact that he transferred between undergraduate colleges, while not uncommon, is notable. Patients with significant NPD often follow a typical pattern of initial success in professional endeavors followed by a fizzling out and withdrawal. This occurs as the individual – often unconsciously – comes to view the job and colleagues as either "unworthy" or alternatively too risky in the sense that the individual may be overshadowed or fail, which would threaten the grandiose sense of self.

The fact that Edward was a polarizing figure during the admissions process is also significant. Individuals with NPD relate to others through idealization or devaluation, both of which can elicit powerful emotional responses. Others who regularly interact with a person with significant narcissistic pathology may, over time, actually assume the idealized or devalued traits assigned to them through the process of projective identification. This appears to have occurred with Professor Wilson who himself adopts an entitled tone when calling the ED to inquire after Edward and who describes other aspects of their interactions over time that suggest some degree of enmeshment in a mutually idealizing relationship with Edward. Notably, these reactions to individuals with NPD are not universal, and the aloof indifference often shown by the narcissistic patient can frequently evoke a reciprocal response – from detached to rageful.

There is a range of severity in NPD. This continuum is common across personality disorders and has been highlighted in the alternative model for personality disorders presented in Section III of the DSM-5. Many individuals with milder NPD symptoms can be remarkably successful in certain aspects of their life, though the diagnosis implies some degree of dysfunction in other areas. It is also common for symptoms to fluctuate in response to life events, as occurs in response to narcissistic injury. Thus, an individual whose narcissism is ordinarily well-preserved and causes minimal disruption may decompensate wildly when a core element of their sense of self (such as their professional success and integrity) is undone. This appears to be the case with Edward. While his narcissistic vulnerability and various maladaptive behaviors were present from the beginning of his time in the lab, it was only in the face of a substantial ego challenge that he unraveled in such a destructive way.

Returning to the details of the case, Edward presented with suicidal behavior and affective disturbance in the setting of multiple negative events consistent with narcissistic injuries. In the ED, Dr. Jensen had been aware of experiencing Edward's suicidality as provocative and feeling initially dismissive of the reports of the circumstances in the apartment and the questionable "suicide text" to Professor Wilson. Dr. Jensen was concerned, however, about the guardedness with which Edward reflected on these circumstances. Moreover, he was careful to keep in mind the elevated risk for suicide in patients with significant narcissistic needs, especially following a situation in which these needs are challenged, as well as the common clinical experience of underestimating the potential for suicide completion in a patient with significant cluster B personality traits – a reaction to negative countertransference responses to the patient's hostile, veiled, or seductive communications. Dr. Jensen made the decision to hospitalize Edward with the goals of further observation and diagnostic clarification, mobilizing social supports, reinforcing ego functioning, providing crisis management in a monitored setting, and planning a safe discharge.

Given his status as a medical student, Edward was transferred and admitted to another hospital not affiliated with his medical school. Edward's care was transferred to Dr. Greene. While Edward had accepted a voluntary admission, his first words to Dr. Greene were "so, I've decided to leave; can you let me know how I can get out of here?" During this initial interview with Dr. Greene, Edward was aloof and condescending, remarking that he understood "you need to protect yourself, so let's go through the motions." He was again minimizing of others' concerns about suicidality. He expressed a belief that his advisor and dean had blown his suicidal behavior out of proportion so that "they can justify removing me." He speculated that they had "freaked out over Anne's ridiculous harassment claims, and they needed a way to make it all go away quietly." When Dr. Greene attempted to challenge some of this logic, Edward would deflect and change the topic.

Edward was very resistant to accepting the role of patient and did not participate in groups or engage in the milieu instead spending time in his room doing crossword puzzles and repeatedly asking the staff for access to a laptop so he could "work on some important data for publication." Given the history of affective dysregulation, Dr. Greene considered treatment with medication. He offered Edward the option of taking a low-dose atypical antipsychotic, explaining that it would target symptoms of anger, but Edward refused.

Supportive psychotherapy may have utility in this setting, but ultimately Dr. Greene's priority was to help Edward and the medical school navigate the current crisis. Given the sensitivity to environmental stressors that individuals with NPD face, it's important to address the relevant circumstances as fully as possible. This is particularly true during high-stake situations (such as potential expulsion from school) where the outcome of the crisis can have significant real-world as well as psychological repercussions. In some ways, the inpatient setting is very well-suited for hosting consequential meetings. Trained mental health clinicians are present and can act as mediators with an eye out for safety concerns. It is also an ideal place for patients in the event they become behaviorally dysregulated, since it is a highly monitored environment designed to preserve safety.

At the time of Edward's admission, the status of the disciplinary response of the medical school was still unknown. With Edward's permission, Dr. Greene was in communication with Professor Wilson and one of the members of the dean's office, who had both called the inpatient team to ask for "a clinical update." Dr. Greene's role in such discussions may seem to place him in a difficult situation. On one hand, Edward is his patient and has afforded him a significant trust in allowing him to speak with the school; Dr. Greene will experience himself as a protector and advocate for his patient. On the other hand, Dr. Greene feels a strong and entirely appropriate sense of responsibility to the profession of medicine, with which Edward's unethical behavior is not aligned. These competing obligations are further complicated by the inherent tendency of the psychiatrist to identify with medical students or doctors, as well as the powerful feelings that individuals with NPD often evoke in clinicians. A variety of countertransference reactions are associated with the treatment of NPD. Among the most common are feelings of being devalued, anger, or boredom. In Edward's case, indignation would be an expected response since Dr. Greene not only resents Edward's aloof condescension but also feels a 'righteous anger' toward a junior member of his profession who has been disrespectful and dishonest. Professor Wilson and the medical school administration are likely to have strong feelings about Edward as well. As a psychiatrist, it will be particularly important for Dr. Greene to recognize and work with these countertransference responses in order to provide the best care to Edward and to ensure optimal and appropriate communication of information with his colleagues at Edward's home school.

Dr. Greene arranged to speak with Professor Wilson and the dean on the telephone. During their conversation, Professor Wilson reported he had found significant problems in his review of Edward's research including evidence that he had altered and falsified certain data. Professor Wilson and the dean expressed guilt that they had not discovered these tendencies earlier in Edward's training and at times seemed to question their own judgment as educators. These reactions likely reflected the lingering effects of Edward's manipulative behavior as well as a non-pathological guilt that one would expect in persons with high conscientiousness. During a pause in the conversation, the dean seemed to blurt out, "we'll have to consider expulsion! He falsified data – the risk is too great, don't you think?" Dr. Greene was not sure if the dean meant that as an explicit question for him but was able to experience it as the dean's expression of validation-seeking in the setting of facing a fraught situation. Without further commenting on the actions that the school would or should take, based on policy and ethos, Dr. Greene felt that it was appropriate for him to validate how complex and problematic the circumstances were and how the responsibilities that the dean and others in the medical school shouldered were weighty.

The next day, Dr. Greene's team was notified that Edward's medical school would be beginning a formal process that could result in expulsion. A concern shared by all involved was the potential risk that Edward might now try to harm himself or strike back at the medical school in some way. Edward has already shown a vulnerability to self-destructive and aggressive behavior in the face of narcissistic injury. For the reasons outlined above, Dr. Greene recommended that this information be shared with Edward while on the inpatient service. Given what he knew about Edward at that point, including how he had responded to the investigation of plagiarism in college, Dr. Greene suspected that Edward would tolerate a departure from medical school much better if he believed that it was actually his decision, or at least felt he had some control in the matter. Dr. Greene explained to the other members of the clinical team that there would be limited value – and significant potential risk – at this early point in treatment in directly challenging Edward's fragile defenses related to his preservation of autonomy and dignity. To be therapeutic, Dr. Greene explained, confrontations and interpretations should be gentle, and are best reserved for modalities with an appropriate frame and therapeutic relationship, such as long-term psychotherapy.

A meeting was arranged on the inpatient unit with Edward, Professor Wilson, the dean, Dr. Greene, and the inpatient social worker. During the meeting, Dr. Greene and the dean explained to Edward that he was under review for expulsion due to the improprieties discovered as well as his egregious behavior toward other students. Edward generally remained silent and aloof throughout. When it was his turn to speak, he replied in a dismissive tone, "I'm not going to work like this. I'm done here."

Edward then turned his attention to Dr. Greene and changed the topic to discharge. Edward implied that his hospitalization had been directed by the medical school "to assuage their guilt over the way they treat students." As he spoke, Edward became increasingly indignant but was regulated enough to walk out of the room rather than engage in further confrontation.

Outcome

Edward remained in good control after the meeting, though he spent the afternoon in his room and declined to speak with the staff who offered to help him process the situation. He was discharged the following day with a plan to return to stay with his parents. Edward had consistently denied suicidal ideation, and there was no evidence of significant manic, depressive, or psychotic symptoms. On the day of discharge, he was superficially cooperative and minimally engaged. He again voiced his displeasure with the medical school and reasserted his intention of leaving. He remained notably externalizing in his responses, emphasizing that the medical school's treatment of him had been "a disgrace" but that he was "going to take the high road" by departing. Dr. Greene offered to provide Edward with a referral for a psychotherapist that might be able to help him "navigate relationships." Edward respectfully declined the offer and was provided with a referral for a clinic near his parents' house.

Afterward, Dr. Greene felt ambivalent about Edward's case and wondered if he could have done more to help. He had approached Edward's care cautiously, avoiding confrontation and overt requests of Edward for self-reflection. He speculated that some of his hesitancy may have been a reflection of the fear and dislike that Edward had evoked in him. At the same time, Dr. Greene was confident that he helped his patient and the medical school navigate a highly charged situation while minimizing disruptive conflict. The immediate ethical violation had been addressed in an appropriate manner. The medical school subsequently developed new policies and procedures to promote research integrity. The final outcome is unsatisfying in that Edward's pathology remains essentially untreated, but the acute preservation of safety and the assistance given to the medical school are no small feats. By speaking with colleagues, Dr. Greene was able to process and reflect on the complex emotional responses that arise when treating a case like this.

Pearls

- Treatment of patients known or suspected to have committed an ethical violation is challenging. Psychiatric diagnoses that may be associated with unethical behavior should be assessed for and addressed. The presence of a psychiatric illness may or may not be a mitigating factor when judging an ethical violation. Support including psychoeducation should be given to administrators or supervisors tasked with responding to the unethical behavior, to the degree that doctor-patient confidentiality permits.
- Narcissistic personality disorder (NPD) occurs across a spectrum of severity, and patients may come to clinical attention for a variety of reasons, including depression, suicidality, or anger. Often, individuals with narcissistic disorders are referred by a third party rather than self-presenting.
- Individuals with NPD are often accomplished and may initially give a favorable impression. They share traits such as perfectionism and aversion to vulnerability which are common among those in the medical field. Medical training similarly frequently tests the fragile defenses of individuals with NPD.

- Psychiatrists treating individuals with NPD are likely to develop strong countertransference responses which may manifest as boredom, defensiveness, or anger. These emotions are likely to be particularly significant when the patient is also a physician.

References

1. American Psychiatric Association. Diagnostic and statistical manual of mental disorders. 5th ed. Arlington: American Psychiatric Publishing; 2013.
2. Bamelis LL, Evers SM, Spinhoven P, Arntz A. Results of a multicenter randomized controlled trial of the clinical effectiveness of schema therapy for personality disorders. Am J Psychiatry. 2014;171:305–22.
3. Kernberg OF. An overview of the treatment of severe narcissistic pathology. Int J Psychoanal. 2014;95:865–88.
4. Ansell EB, Wright AG, Markowitz JC, Sanislow CA, Hopwood CJ, Zanarini MC, Yen S, Pinto A, McGlashan TH, Grilo CM. Personality disorder risk factors for suicide attempts over 10 years of follow-up. Personal Disord. 2015;6:161–7.
5. Yen S, Pagano ME, Shea MT, Grilo CM, Gunderson JG, Skodol AE, McGlashan TH, Sanislow CA, Bender DS, Zanarini MC. Recent life events preceding suicide attempts in a personality disorder sample: findings from the collaborative longitudinal personality disorders study. J Consult Clin Psychol. 2005;73:99–105.

Suggested Reading

Caligor E, Levy KN, Yeomans FE. Narcissistic personality disorder: diagnostic and clinical challenges. Am J Psychiatry. 2015;172:415–22.
Gabbard GO. Transference and countertransference: developments in the treatment of narcissistic personality disorder. Psychiatr Ann. 2009;39:129–36.

Chapter 19
The Case of Owen Burt: Running on Empty

Janna S. Gordon-Elliott

Case

Owen Burt is a 36-year-old internist working in a busy academic medical center who comes to see Dr. Agni, a psychiatrist in his institution, for a chief complaint of "I don't know, I just can't cope, I must be depressed."

Owen works as an inpatient medicine attending on a general medicine service, where he supervises residents and physician assistants and provides direct patient care. He graduated residency in internal medicine at age 29 having gone straight through from college to medical school and then residency. He chose not to do a fellowship and instead took a job as a supervising attending in the residents' clinic, hoping to spend a few years making money to pay off loans. After 4 years, feeling unstimulated by the work and bothered by feelings of resenting some of his patients for "noncompliance," he decided to shift into inpatient work, where the plan was to spend alternating periods doing inpatient medicine and working on an academic project. He initially was invigorated by the change, remembering the "fun frenzy" of acute care

J. S. Gordon-Elliott, MD (✉)
Weill Cornell Medical College/New York-Presbyterian Hospital,
New York, NY, USA
e-mail: jsg2005@med.cornell.edu

© Springer Nature Switzerland AG 2019   223
J. S. Gordon-Elliott, A. H. Rosen (eds.), *Early Career Physician Mental Health and Wellness*,
https://doi.org/10.1007/978-3-030-10952-3_19

work and the team approach to patient care. Three months into the new job, he was asked to cover the inpatient service for a few months longer before getting a month for academic time, because of an acute staffing issue. He realized he was somewhat relieved to do this, feeling "spooked" by the thought of starting a project – "how would I know what project to choose?" Over the next 3 years, it seemed to him that there was always a "coverage issue." Having not identified a major area for academic focus, he continued to either volunteer or be asked to provide clinical coverage. He rarely took vacations; he was encouraged to use his vacation time, but when he tried to find a week to take off, there "always seemed to be conflicts" with other people's schedule. He found himself staying late most days finishing "endless notes and paperwork." He thought about going to his peers or his division chief to talk about the sense of clinical and administrative burden but figured "it must be my problem – I'm just not efficient enough." He was noticing over time less interest in his patients. He resented new admissions and felt "uninterested" in patients. He would find himself feeling anxious before a month when he was assigned to supervise the resident service (as opposed to the service staffed with physician assistants), realizing that he was finding it hard to "get excited" about "the same old, same old," and feeling uneasy about keeping up to date on the literature and engaging the residents on educational topics. He felt less anxious with the physician assistants but also found himself "really frustrated" with them – describing a sense of needing to "micromanage everything" because many of them were very new to the job. He explained that they didn't seem to be able to "problem-solve" effectively, so he began just giving them "to do lists" rather than encouraging them to come up with their own plans.

In his personal life, he had moved into a one-bedroom apartment without a roommate after his first year in the ambulatory clinic. He noticed how his friend network had seemed to "shrink" since then. He told Dr. Agni that he used to enjoy team sports, playing in a basketball league through residency and his first few years afterward but that he had stopped going because "it was too hard to be sure I could get out of work on time." He admitted that during residency this was an issue, too, but that he would be active in the league when on quieter rotations and pull back during busier times. Now, he felt like there was too much of a "hill to climb" to start and stop like that, and now it felt easier to "just not go." Much of his social life had revolved around his basketball friends, and now he was seeing those friends infrequently – "I guess I just lost that connection; maybe they weren't really my friends, anyway."

On more review of his life and history, Owen denied any history of psychiatric issues. He is the eldest of three children; his father is an endocrinologist, and his mother is a lawyer working in the public sector. He reported that he first wanted to become a physician "at age 3," describing memories of his father allowing him to listen to heart sounds with his stethoscope. When he was 11, his grandmother had a stroke, and, though his younger siblings would express not wanting to go visit her in the rehab center while she was recovering, he recalled feeling "comfortable" sitting with her – helping her "learn her words again" and watching her work with the physical therapists. He said that some of this may also have been related to his "being the good kid – the one who helped and did what was expected… that's who I was, still am?." Medical school had been pleasurable but stressful. He noticed feeling very competitive with his classmates in a way he hadn't noticed in school settings before. He struggled with learning the volume of material he had to master, trying to use the study habits that had thus far served him well, but that now were seemingly taking too much time, such that he would frequently only be able to review half the material before an exam. He was assigned a tutor, which he found "insulting," and recalled feeling like he was being told he needed to do it "her way, not my way." He gradually learned a system that was more efficient, and he scored adequately well on his tests. He felt like he hit his stride in the clerkships, where he enjoyed the patient contact, found it easier to study the material because of the clinical context, and "got along with the attendings."

Coming back to the present day, Owen reported that 2 months ago he had experienced a "bad event." He had a busy service, though described most of their medical issues as "low acuity." One day, he was called by the hospital pharmacy because he had placed an order for a medication at ten times the appropriate dose. The medication had not been dispensed, as the pharmacy caught the aberrant order. He remembered being "horrified" by this, wondering how he could have made that mistake. That evening, while walking down the hallway of the inpatient ward on his way out of the hospital, he heard loud gasps coming from a patient's room. Inside, he saw the patient for whom he had earlier written the mistakened order lying in bed, appearing panicked and apparently unable to breathe. Owen reported that "from there, it's all a little fuzzy." He ran to the bedside and tried to press the call button to get the nurses' attention. He felt like he kept pressing it over and over and nothing was happening. He then stood over the patient's bed "just staring at her." A nurse walked by and saw the patient and called a code. Staff rushed into the room and the code team arrived and took over. He recalled standing there feeling "frozen" and "useless." He could not sleep that night and continued to have difficulties falling asleep for several nights afterward. He did not understand why he "froze" like that; he knew how to function in emergencies. He knew the patient had not received the mistakened medication order, and she was not known to have respiratory issues; so he could "rationally" understand he didn't miss anything, but he could not stop worrying. He felt "ashamed" about being found by the nurse "not doing anything."

Since then, he has been having initial insomnia two or three times a week and has found himself worrying about patients and "mistakes." He has felt "anxious and uncomfortable" with patients – doubting his ability to take care of them. He admitted, however, that he had been feeling different "for a while, maybe months." He felt like the clinical work never ended and that he could never catch up. His eating, which he used to monitor because of his basketball playing, had become more "erratic." His weight was the same, but he was often skipping meals and then eating "junk because I know I'm supposed to eat something." He admitted to feeling more irritable. His energy was low. He admitted that he had been going "from home to work to home to work" with few social activities or other breaks in the monotony. He denied significant alcohol use or other substance use. He denied thoughts of death or suicide.

Dr. Agni listened and found herself thinking about her own experience 5 years before in a previous job. She had worked in an outpatient clinic where there was "constant understaffing" and "one new administrative headache added on top of another on top of another." She felt "burned out" and asked for support and felt that "no one listened." She eventually felt all she could do was quit, which she did. She had some savings and decided to not press herself to find a new job immediately. She reengaged with a previous therapist and started with twice weekly dynamic therapy. She spent 2 years doing per diem shifts at a couple of local clinics in order to make ends meet. She felt unsatisfied and angry at her previous employer. At the time of meeting Owen, she had been in her current position for the past year and was enjoying it. She had a lot of responsibilities but found the work stimulating and generally liked her administration and peers.

With 10 minutes left in the session, after listening to Owen and asking clarifying questions, Dr. Agni said to Owen that it seemed he was in a "difficult position" and that it must be "hard" to be "never given a break." She said that she recommended he come back next week and that they could talk about ways to make things better – "even if that means leaving your job." She also said that sometimes patients can get help by understanding themselves better, and they could talk about possibly starting psychodynamic psychotherapy. They made an appointment for the following week.

Principles of Diagnosis and Management

Diagnosis

The preferred diagnosis for Owen from the perspective of the *Diagnostic and Statistical Manual of Mental Disorders*, Fifth Edition (DSM-5), is adjustment disorder with depressed mood [1]. Owen has symptoms of mood changes, including low mood and irritability, with sleep disturbance, feelings of lower energy/listlessness, and a decrease both in his sense of self-worth and value and in his general experience of pleasure from life, all in the context of what he describes as chronic stress related to his work as well as a recent distressing experience involving clinical care. Major depressive disorder (MDD) should be considered, too, with Owen responding affirmatively several of the diagnostic symptoms. When implementing DSM criteria, however, it is important to draw on clinical experience and judgment, ultimately basing the assessment on the presenting features within the context of the quality of the patient's presentation (on exam and in how the patient describes symptoms) and the situation.

Owen's presentation could represent posttraumatic stress disorder (PTSD, also reviewed previously in Chaps. 5 and 9 of this book). PTSD, in the Trauma and Stressor-Related Disorder category along with adjustment disorder, develops in response to a traumatic event and is characterized by intrusion symptoms, persistent avoidance, changes in mood or cognitions, and alterations in arousal. Owen witnessed and was involved in a critical incident at work in which – though not outside of the range of what a physician might expect to encounter in high-acuity settings, like the hospital – he experienced as particularly frightening and distressing. There is a literature to support the development of PTSD among healthcare workers [2]. Owen's reported sense of feeling disconnected from his work and patients could be an avoidance symptom, and his low mood, irritability, and impaired sense of self-efficacy and self-worth could similarly reflect features of PTSD (negative alterations of mood and cognition and/or altered arousal). It may be that an emerging depressive syndrome prior to the event put him at higher risk for experiencing the event as especially traumatic.

Obsessive compulsive personality disorder (OCPD), characterized by a preoccupation with control, order, and perfectionism, to an excessive degree, leading to distress of impairment in functioning, is also on the differential diagnosis. Traits of OCPD are common in physicians, as many of these traits can be highly adaptive, either in isolation or in limited contexts. High conscientiousness, attention to detail, and striving for excellence are all features we would look for in a healthcare provider. When such traits are pervasive or extreme, they can become more problematic. Individuals may have difficulty delegating tasks due to a belief that no one else could perform the task as precisely and thus become overburdened, resentful, and even ineffective. Interpersonal rigidity may make it hard to work with these individuals – as their colleague, supervisor, or patient. It is appropriate (and important) for Owen to be concerned about his performance and potential for medical mistakes; it is possible that – in the context of OCPD or traits of OCPD – he has a tendency to overestimate the impact of his actions, both good and bad, thus becoming overly self-critical in the setting of negative or uncertain outcomes. Some of what he reports in the interpersonal sphere could reflect characteristic ways in which he engages with others (i.e., tendency to overmanage those he supervises, avoidance of authority figures out of concern for being criticized, minimizing the benefit he might get from asking for others' help). More information about his behavior and relationships over his life, if revealing a pervasive pattern of OCPD traits and consistent functional difficulties, could support this diagnosis while being cautious about assigning a personality disorder diagnosis in the setting of an active depressive or adjustment disorder, which may exacerbate existing personality traits.

Alcohol use, or another substance use disorder, should be assessed for, given the presence of mood disturbance, a possible lapse of judgment at work, and sleep changes. Owen is denying excessive alcohol use, and the history does not describe past issues with substance misuse. Depending on the degree of suspicion, further assessment, including use of self- or clinician-administered screening tools, or toxicology assays may be considered.

Dr. Agni documented in her notes that the DSM-5 diagnosis that fit the best was adjustment disorder with depressed mood, though her assessment was that Owen was experiencing *burnout*. Burnout is a syndrome, most commonly examined within the context of a work situation, that presents with a range of mental and physical complaints and has been defined by the core features of emotional exhaustion, depersonalization, and reduction in one's sense of personal accomplishment [3, 4]. All three of these characteristic symptom clusters may not always be present. A physician with burnout may describe feeling emotionally depleted or "spent," with "nothing left to give"; overwhelmed or "unable to keep my head above water"; detached from patients, "unempathic." or cynical; and unsatisfied by work, ineffective or "failing" at work, or distressed by the "meaninglessness" or "pointlessness" of work.

The implications of burnout in medicine are substantial. Those with burnout appear to have a higher risk for poor mental and physical health outcomes, including the development of depression, substance use, and suicidal ideation, as well as poor self-care (including reduced attention to one's physical needs and preventive care). Physicians with burnout are more likely to leave clinical medicine at some point in their career. Burnout may negatively impact the individual's relationships with colleagues and loved ones. It has been shown to be associated with impaired patient care, including an increase in medical errors and reduced patient satisfaction. On a systems level, burnout may lead to loss of clinical productivity, attrition the workforce, reduced access to care, and increased healthcare costs [4].

Burnout can exist at any point during one's medical career. Once thought to be a condition primarily affecting physicians after an accumulation of many years of practice, burnout may, in fact, be more common at earlier stages and is notably prevalent among trainees, with half of medical students demonstrating symptoms, or the full syndrome, of burnout and with rates that rise over residency [3].

Drivers of burnout include those factors, both personal and institutional- or system-based, that appear to precipitate burnout. Individuals may also have specific vulnerability to burnout due to personal features that put them more at risk. Drivers related to the institution or healthcare system include, but are not limited to, excessive workload; clerical demands (e.g., high documentation requirements in the electronic health record) and deficiencies in support for such administrative tasks; impaired integration of life in and out of work (e.g., work requirements excessively preventing adequate attention to other aspects of life; demands requiring a surplus of work to be done from home, such as note-writing; or inflexibility of the system not allowing for opportunities to handle some aspects of work from home if that would allow for more time with family or in activities that promote recovery or life fulfillment); and excessive systems-based demands that lessen the physician's sense of autonomy in work. Personal factors may include limited social support or high-stress personal issues and educational debt. Aspects specific to the individual that have some evidence for increasing the risk for burnout include female gender, nonminority status, personality traits such as high being highly self-critical, and tendencies to not prioritize self-care [3–5]. Burnout may also be "contagious"; exposure to supervisors with burnout may impact the well-being and even the burnout incidence among trainees [3]. Importantly, the prevailing perspective is that systems-based factors are stronger drivers of burnout than are individual-based factors.

Management and Treatment

Adjustment disorder with depressed mood and major depressive disorder both present with low mood, commonly with some degree of inflexible thinking (e.g., tendency to interpret events in a critical or pessimistic way, to dwell over personal deficiencies, to have difficulty achieving and maintaining a hopeful outlook). Adjustment disorder is, by definition, considered to develop in response to an adverse experience or situation, while MDD is frequently precipitated or perpetuated by life stressors. Both disorders may be treated with psychotherapy that targets underlying psychological processes that contribute to the development and maintenance of the symptoms. Cognitive behavioral therapy (CBT) will address maladaptive thinking styles that drive mood and behavior. Psychodynamic psychotherapy will encourage exploration of long-standing patterns of interpersonal relatedness and one's sense of oneself and others that may increase vulnerability to depressive responses to certain stressors. Supportive psychotherapy will reinforce the patient's adaptive coping mechanisms while proving a safe space to assess, and come up with solutions for, current challenges. Interpersonal therapy will focus on the characteristic ways in which the individual engages with others, making explicit connections to the depression the patient is experiencing; identifying ways to communicate needs more effectively and find satisfaction in relationships is viewed as a means to promote emotional health and treat the depression. Pharmacotherapy, most commonly antidepressants, may be combined with psychotherapy or used alone, depending on factors such as severity of symptoms, patient preference, and access to skilled providers for psychological treatment.

The treatment of PTSD, as outlined in more detail in Chaps. 5 and 9, may involve CBT and other forms of psychotherapy. Medications, including antidepressants and adrenergic system modulators, may be utilized.

Patients with OCPD will not necessarily present for treatment, as insight into one's problematic patterns may be limited. Some may seek care for help to manage distress related to what is experienced as "other people's" problems; some may come to attention due to pressure from others – including spouses, friends, or authorities – because of difficulties arising as a result of the person's negative behavior patterns.

Treatment may start with nonjudgmental examination of common themes in one's life, identification of one's agency in the situations that are causing problems or distress, and gentle examination of rigidly held assumptions and preferences, with the goal of gaining more insight and a wider array of perspectives about, and responses to, one's environment.

The management of burnout is a topic of significant interest, with a new, but expanding, supporting literature. Strategies for preventing and addressing burnout can be categorized as either coming from the organizational- or system-level and those focused on the individual. Organizational-based strategies may include duty-hour limits (the institution of the 80-hour workweek for residents appears to have been associated with reduction of burnout), creative ways to enhance flexibility for work-home conflicts, physician involvement in establishing of administrative processes as they relate to clinical care, and development of wellness programs with top-down institutional support and ratification. Individual-focused strategies may include wellness activities, such as mindfulness, healthy lifestyle practices, and enhancing one's social supports [3, 4, 6]. In general, given the evidence that institution-based factors are the primary drivers of burnout, it is important to address those issues when working with a patient with burnout symptoms; focusing entirely on individual factors will not only miss opportunities to modify the situation leading to burnout but also has a significant chance of making the patient feel "to blame for getting burned out" rather than to see oneself an individual who, due to a combination of institutional and personal factors, was vulnerable to developing the burnout syndrome. The meaning of these two messages is clearly very different and important to explicitly state, without overemphasizing either of the two "sides."

Finding ways to encourage *joy* in one's work – reengaging in the ideas or activities that originally motivated the decision to become a physician, taking pleasure in interactions with patients, noticing aspects of each day to be grateful for – is being emphasized by experts as part of a broad effort to reduce burnout among physicians and trainees.

Principles for Doctors Treating Doctors

Health has been defined by the World Health Organization as "a state of complete physical, mental, and social well-being, and not merely the absence of disease or infirmity" [7]. The National Wellness Institute later described *wellness* as "a conscious, self-directed and evolving process of achieving full potential" [8]. There are many elements or *pillars* of wellness, dividing wellness into its essential components: emotional, spiritual, social, environmental, intellectual, occupational, physical, and financial [9].

Wellness is not something that is achieved; rather, it is a dynamic process of continuing attention to oneself and one's environment and adaptations that promote a fulfilling existence. A core aspect of wellness is resilience to the various stressors of life – unavoidable and, in fact, necessary features of life that influence, shape, and strengthen us. Resilience involves the capacity to be flexible in the face of new situations and pressures and some degree of reserve that can be tapped into during taxing times. Just like having savings in a bank account to cover for events that are not directly budgeted for, but that predictably will arise, we benefit from emotional and physical resources that can be drawn from when our output exceeds our input. For example, prioritizing a healthy amount of sleep most of the time allows our bodies to withstand brief bouts of limited sleep due to a period of abnormally high workload. Similarly, addressing our emotional well-being with loving relationships, engagement in pleasurable activities, and attention to our psychological needs, as well as adequate management of any psychiatric conditions present, can keep us sturdy in the face of a short stretch of acute stress following a life disappointment or loss.

When stress is more enduring, unpredictable, or seemingly out of one's control, it can begin to deplete personal reserves. Over time, this can lead to a state of bare subsistence – simply getting by, or surviving, rather than thriving. In such a state, mood and interpersonal relationships may suffer, self-care may be neglected, and maladaptive behaviors, such as substance use, may develop. Empathy diminishes; generosity feels like a burden. Burnout is an extreme consequence for the individual exposed to uninterrupted stress with low perceived personal control and high external demands. All occupations, given the right circumstances, can promote burnout. Other situations, such as caring for an ailing loved one, can have the same effect. It is not surprising that medicine is a profession in which burnout is prevalent, due to the high stakes of the work (often life or death or equally acute), the substantial needs of clients (i.e., patients and families), and the complexities of the healthcare system which can constrain one's options and autonomy. Add to this the long work-hours, financial debt, and years of training, as well as personal factors that can be common among physicians, such as exacting standards for oneself, and high capacity for delay of gratification: a potential recipe for burnout without the right checks in place to prevent it.

In addition to the strategies mentioned earlier in *Management and Treatment*, which have been studied and shown to have some efficacy in minimizing and addressing burnout, individual and systems can take actions to increase resilience to stress. Diversification of one's sources of meaning, self-worth, and satisfaction – for example, identifying not only as a skilled physician but as a good friend to others, a talented writer, and even a snappy dresser – can allow one to continue to feel competent and valuable even when one area of life (e.g., one's relationship to one's work) is temporarily suffering. Active seeking of joyful moments and gratitude in one's relationships, hobbies, environment, and work can raise one's threshold for stress, struggle, and frustration. Self-awareness, which may be sought through meaningful relationships, self-reflection, athletic pursuits, spirituality, and psychotherapy (among others) can allow for identification of one's personal pitfalls, emotional triggers, and warning signs – with the result of less depletion and harm and more recovery and growth.

Dr. Owen Burt presented to Dr. Agni with concerns that he was "depressed." He was experiencing mood changes, doubts about his efficacy and capability in his work, and a general sense of emotional and physical depletion. Dr. Agni, due to her own experiences with burnout and her awareness of its general prevalence in the healthcare profession, puts effort into exploring the quality and form of Owen's symptoms to better differentiate a burnout syndrome from other major psychiatric issues, with special attention to the overlap between burnout and a major depressive episode (see Fig. 19.1). While the two syndromes have many common features and common risk factors and may coexist, and each predisposes to the development of the other, they are distinct and may present independently.

To begin exploring this overlap, it is important to consider the *stress response* – sympathetic overdrive related to an experienced stressful experience through activation of networks in the brain and body, including the hypothalamic-pituitary-adrenal (HPA) axis. While this response is adaptive

Features of MDE	Presentation in Burnout
- Low/depressed mood	• Emotional exhaustion, less pleasure and satisfaction from work, reduced personal accomplishment +/- feelings of inefficacy at work
- Diminished interest or pleasure	• Symptoms described as related to work • May extend to other areas of life as burnout syndrome progresses
- Feelings of worthlessness/guilt	• When imagining being free of work-related burdens, can imagine reduction or elimination of these symptoms
- Changes in sleep - Changes in eating - Fatigue	• May be present as part of the stress response • Related to the emotional and physiologic stress of work • Prioritizing work and others' needs over one's own
- Changes in concentration - Restlessness or feeling slowed	• May be present as part of the stress response
- Thoughts of death, suicidality	• If present, consider other diagnoses, including MDD

FIGURE 19.1 Relationship between features of a major depressive episode and burnout

in situations of acute danger or risk, chronic activation due to one's experience of ongoing threat or stress can lead to a prolonged state of HPA hyperactivity, with impact on cognitive, physical, and emotional well-being. The way different individuals perceive and process stressful triggers that are not acutely life-threatening (such as workload pressures, concerns about performance/evaluation, emotional intensity of the work setting) will influence the development of the stress response – with those individuals who feel less able to cope and less resilient or who engage in maladaptive behaviors as a result (such as substance use, poor self-care), being at higher risk for chronic activation of stress response than those with more adaptive coping and reactions to the stressful situations.

An individual with burnout may have some of the core physical symptoms of a MDE, such as sleep disturbance, poor energy, and eating and weight changes, as a result of remaining in a chronic state of the stress response. Additionally, in burnout, the enduring nature of stress and demoralization can manifest, as described, with de-prioritization of one's own needs, which may lead to poor attention to functions such as sleep, nutrition, exercise, and emotional "recovery" time, which can all contribute to these physical symptoms. It can be difficult to differentiate the syndromes when assessing these symptoms. It may be useful – if relevant – to ask about these physical symptoms during a recent period of time away from work for more than a few days (e.g., a vacation), to see if there was improvement in these symptoms during that time, in which case the clinician might consider burnout over MDE. Owen explained to Dr. Agni that he had not had more than 3 days off of work for the past several months due to the coverage schedule and his own admitted "failure to just schedule a vacation – I just haven't felt like I can." Dr. Agni knew that evaluating these symptoms based on a single-day or weekend off may not be an adequate test, as it may take longer for the stress response and emotional experience of work to dissipate enough for these physical functions to begin to re-equilibrate.

The cognitive/emotional features of a MDE, including depressed mood, anhedonia, and thoughts of self-worth, may be worth assessing more closely to help differentiate between the syndromes. In burnout, the changes in these areas have the quality of being explicitly tied to the work situation, with the ability to feel improved mood, more pleasure, and more self-worth in other settings. Not uncommonly, the burnout syndrome is substantial enough that the individual feels so depleted at work that these features extend to other areas of life. Owen described to Dr. Agni a sense of having "nothing left to give" to his loved ones and friends, even on the weekends. "I tell myself, you have a whole day off – you should go do something fun, but I just can't." Still aware of how burnout symptoms can begin to affect all areas of life, Dr. Agni asked Owen a theoretical question: *what if I could magically tell you that all these burdens have been lifted off your shoulders? You can rest for the next few weeks, you don't have to come back to this specific job, you have time and resources to recover and think about what you want to do next. How would that feel?* Owen's response was quite typical of burnout. His physical demeanor softened. His shoulders dropped; he looked momentarily sad but then looked up for the first time in several minutes and made eye contact and appeared to take the first full breath that Dr. Agni had seen him take so far during their meeting. He said that this would feel like a "total relief. I know it's not possible, but I just can't figure out another way around this mountain." A theoretical question like this allows the clinician to explore the breadth of the symptoms. In burnout, though the symptoms may extend past the work situation, they are intricately linked to the presence of the work-related stressors; therefore, considering ways to improve the situation, or even make it "disappear," can allow the patient to demonstrate a very different thinking style and outlook. On the other hand, in an active MDE, such symptoms tend to be pervasive and not flexible – the patient's perspective remains bleak and without potential for improvement.

Suicidality is a feature of depression as well as other psychiatric disorders. When present, the clinician should be considering depression or other disorders instead of, or in addition to, burnout. Whether or not burnout is thought to be the primary issue, suicidality should be taken as a potential acute risk and should trigger a full safety assessment and safety management plan. Owen consistently denied suicidal ideation or significant thoughts of death.

Dr. Agni had knowledge and experience to help guide her assessment of burnout in Owen. In addition to the tricky differentiation between burnout and depression, other obstacles interfere with appropriate assessment of burnout. To start, the symptoms of burnout in a physician can be easy to miss. During an assessment, the psychiatrist, especially if it is the first time meeting the patient, might view some of the described symptoms as "normal trait characteristics" of a physician (e.g., obsessionality, difficulty delegating, feeling "stressed"), as well as simply part of the "cost of doing business" of being a physician (e.g., high workload, sleep deprivation, not always being able to prioritize self-care). The assessing physician's internalized pride in the suffering or burdens related to being in medicine – a cognitive bias that is largely unconscious and shared by many physicians – may lead to missing burnout. Pervasive beliefs among physicians that are deeply woven within the fabric of the medical culture and training experience, such as "I've done this, I'm stronger for it" and "we're all anxious, easily stressed people," may be present as the physician-assessor evaluates the physician-patient with burnout. While this tendency to normalize is usually unintentional or well-intentioned, it may prevent recognizing clinically meaningful symptoms of burnout. Data show that medical students start training no more vulnerable to burnout than their peers and yet develop relatively higher rates of burnout over the training period [3]. It is essential that burnout symptoms not be quickly dismissed as related to "the physician personality" or experience.

These cognitive- and emotionally based perspectives and biases, among other countertransference experiences, will influence the psychiatrist's assessment of the physician-patient with burnout. Not uncommonly, a negative countertransference may develop in which the patient is viewed as "weak" for not being able to "withstand" the pressures of medicine; this may lead to missing the burnout diagnosis but also to offering unhelpful responses to the patient – from subtle devaluing comments, even if meant supportively (e.g., "you'll be ok, this is just part of the job!"), to more explicit criticism (e.g., over-valuing the perspective, or even "taking the side," of the authority figures in the story that the patient relates), to not offering the patient appropriate treatment, and to even missing acute danger (e.g., not asking about suicidality or risky behaviors).

Dr. Agni, though attuned to burnout, fell into some minor traps with Owen based on her residual unprocessed responses to her own experience and her difficulty identifying related countertransference themes. She took the time to assess for burnout but then went immediately into a plan of action. In so doing, she missed opportunities to allow Owen to feel validated and heard, and she came up with a plan not attuned to Owen's specific needs but one that was (we assume) based more on her own approach to burnout 5 years before. Her ongoing disgruntlement related to her experience in her prior job led her to not be able to fully place herself in Owen's position – to learn enough about his specific needs and experiences and what might help him. She may have jumped to solutions such as leaving the job (something that Owen may, in fact, eventually decide to do but an option that would not ideally be an immediate option without further exploration), rather than explicitly facilitating Owen's exploration of the areas of his current situation that seem unmanageable, potential areas for improvement, and his overall goals. She appropriately asked him the theoretical question about how he would think and feel if the situation was "eliminated." In some situations, it may also be helpful to directly mention leaving the job as one of the many possibilities; this may be useful if the patient is feeling particularly "trapped" or over-burdened by projected judgment from others. Similarly, Dr. Agni outlined a treatment plan prematurely that echoed her own process to recover from burnout (including her recommendation for dynamic psychotherapy). For Owen, other equally appropriate treatment options might be considered, such as mindfulness training (see Chap. 20 for more information), consideration of a brief medical leave, or addressing institutional changes that could improve his situation. Even working with Owen to problem-solve over finding a way to schedule a week-long vacation in the next few weeks might be an initial intervention that could help him feel empowered and more hopeful and serve as a good start in addressing his burnout syndrome, as well as engaging him in care. Minor missteps like these by the psychiatrist can be repaired but would ideally be ones that could be avoided with careful attention to the patient and to countertransference experiences. More serious mistakes, such as not doing a full safety assessment or behaving in more explicitly devaluing way with the patient, may not be able to be recovered from or may put the patient at risk.

Outcome

Owen came back the following week. He was quiet at the start and Dr. Agni allowed for a period of silence. She had been reflecting on their session the previous week and realized that she had felt uncharacteristically "fervent" during the session. She later realized that she was activated by her frustrations about her own experience in her last job and felt "excited to fix Owen's problem." She even identified a desire in herself to "rally him" against the institution. She realized this had played out with her not spending as much time eliciting his thoughts about the situation and what might help, as well as offering solutions before she "really knew what was going on." After a minute of quiet, she decided to ask Owen if he had thoughts about their meeting or if anything had occurred to him over the week that he had not mentioned. He looked up and said that he had initially felt "a lot of relief" during the session – "like, maybe it wasn't my fault" – but admitted that after leaving the office, he felt "just as hopeless" and "uncertain." Dr. Agni told him she wondered if it might be helpful to write a list of the issues that Owen considered his priorities and another list of the aspects of his work and life that he felt were either problems or interfering with his priorities. He said this sounded like a good idea – "I feel so jumbled up, it's like my brain is spinning." Over that session, Dr. Agni mostly listened to Owen, offering some assistance in putting words to his thoughts while checking in frequently about whether he felt she was "on target." She suggested they meet the following week to continue the process. Over the next few meetings, they strategized for Owen to take a week of vacation at the start of his upcoming academic period. They went over various potential solutions – from going on medical leave, to finding an academic project that would bring him "excitement and joy" and getting a mentor to help him with it, to consulting a career coach to consider other job options. Dr. Agni repeatedly said that none of these options were better or worse, and they were also not mutually exclusive. Owen expressed feeling less "trapped" and more "hopeful."

After Owen returned from his vacation, they made a plan for him to schedule a meeting with his division chief to discuss his role and his career goals. They talked about ways for Owen to advocate for structural changes in how his and the other inpatient attendings' schedule and workflow were organized. He became excited talking about this, realizing this might be a meaningful quality improvement project for him to work on, with mentorship, as his academic project. He had seen a flyer about a "burnout prevention" lecture being given to the residents and decided he would go to that to hear more about what the hospital was providing for residents in this area. Significant current attention to medical trainee wellness, promoted by organizing bodies such as the Liaison Committee on Medical Education (LCME) and Accreditation Council for Graduate Medical Education (ACGME), is allowing for development of more direct efforts to manage and prevent burnout among students and residents. Those out of training may find fewer resources or less attention to burnout in their work environments and may be at increased risk of not having burnout identified until it becomes more severe or problematic. Dr. Agni supported Owen's idea about a quality project related to burnout, seeing this as a way for Owen to feel more confident and to enhance his agency in improving his situation, as well as a meaningful contribution to his division.

Owen was sleeping better, getting exercise more regularly, and finding himself looking forward to evenings out with friends. He reported enjoying patient encounters more and not feeling dread before work. He talked about his thoughts for the future, not sure what path he might end up taking but "open to possibilities." Dr. Agni noticed that she, too, was feeling different. She felt a renewed faith in the hospital system and in the resilience of her colleagues. She wrote a personal essay about her experience with personal burnout and helping others manage burnout and submitted it for electronic publication to a physician-centered national website. It was accepted.

Pearls
- Burnout is a syndrome characterized by emotional exhaustion, depersonalization, and a reduced sense of personal accomplishment and may develop in the context of a work situation where there is a combination of low perceived autonomy and intense external demands.
- Management of burnout will need to address both the organization-level and individual-level drivers of burnout.
- Burnout may share many features with psychiatric disorders, including depression, and may coexist with other disorders, necessitating a careful assessment.
- Beliefs and attitudes about the physician experience may influence the psychiatrist's assessment of burnout in another physician.

References

1. American Psychiatric Association. Diagnostic and statistical manual of mental disorders. 5th ed. Arlington: American Psychiatric Publishing; 2013.
2. de Boer J, Lok A, Van't Verlaat E, Duivenvoorden HJ, Bakker AB, Smit BJ. Work-related critical incidents in hospital-based health care providers and the risk of post-traumatic stress symptoms, anxiety, and depression: a meta-analysis. Soc Sci Med. 2011;73:316–26.
3. Dyrbye L, Shanafelt T. A narrative review on burnout experienced by medical students and residents. Med Educ. 2016;50:132–49.
4. West CP, Dyrbye LN, Shanafelt TD. Physician burnout: contributors, consequences and solutions. J Intern Med. 2018;283:516–29.
5. Patel RS, Bachu R, Adikey A, Malik M, Shah M. Factors related to physician burnout and its consequences: a review. Behav Sci. 2018;8:98–104.
6. Busireddy KR, Miller JA, Ellison K, Ren V, Qayyum R, Panda M. Efficacy of interventions to reduce resident physician burnout: a systematic review. J Grad Med Educ. 2017;9:294–301.
7. Constitution of the World Health Organization. 1946. https://www.who.int/about/mission/en/. Accessed 23 Nov 2018.
8. National Wellness Institute. https://www.nationalwellness.org/page/AboutWellness. Accessed 20 Nov 2018.
9. Substance Abuse and Mental Health Services Organization. https://www.samhsa.gov/wellness-initiative/eight-dimensions-wellness. Accessed 20 Nov 2018.

Suggested Reading

Messias E, Flynn V. The tired, retired, and recovered physician: professional burnout versus major depressive disorder. Am J Psychiatry. 2018;175:716–9.
West CP, Dyrbye LN, Erwin PJ, Shanafelt TD. Interventions to prevent and reduce physician burnout: a systematic review and meta-analysis. Lancet. 2016;388:2272–81.

Chapter 20
The Case of Jerome Ocean: A Student's Classic Conundrum

Christopher R. Green and Janna S. Gordon-Elliott

Case

Jerome Ocean, a 23-year-old man enrolled in his second year of medical school, presented to a student mental health clinic for an evaluation by a senior psychiatrist, Dr. Stone, presenting with a chief complaint of, "I think I have GAD, and I'm really worried my panic attacks are going to get in the way of my clerkship performance." He described feeling like he was "worrying all the time," and he reported incidents of acute escalation of anxiety and physical symptoms of arousal in clinical settings.

In gathering history, Dr. Stone learned that this was the first time Jerome had sought psychiatric treatment or even felt like he might need to see a psychiatrist. He had been brought up by "down-to-earth, Midwestern parents" and had a "busy but happy childhood," though later revealed that at age ten he had lost his father in a car accident, leading to a

C. R. Green, MD · J. S. Gordon-Elliott, MD (✉)
Weill Cornell Medical College/New York-Presbyterian Hospital, New York, NY, USA
e-mail: crg9026@nyp.org; jsg2005@med.cornell.edu

© Springer Nature Switzerland AG 2019
J. S. Gordon-Elliott, A. H. Rosen (eds.), *Early Career Physician Mental Health and Wellness*,
https://doi.org/10.1007/978-3-030-10952-3_20

period of mourning. Jerome was successful both at school and in helping out his mother as she struggled with the punctuated course of her multiple sclerosis. On occasion, he would reflect on his longing for a father but believed he was strong enough to "make it through." He was accepted to a flagship state school an hour drive from home and majored in biology with excellent grades. He had some "normal anxiety" about exams and would often spend long nights studying so that he could get into medical school. His goal was to become a neurologist and take care of patients with conditions like his mother's. During college, Jerome visited her once or twice a month to "help out around the house." He managed to have a good social life, with several close friends and two long-term romantic relationships. Initially, he thought he would continue on his expected path by going to the medical school attached to his university and was indeed accepted there. His plans slowly changed after he was accepted to a top medical school on the West Coast. He had trouble recalling whether it was he or his mother who had decided, but they came to an understanding that he would attend the private school. "There was a bit of guilt" and anxiety about who would take care of his mother, but she encouraged him not to miss out on the golden opportunity.

These feelings dissipated when he actually matriculated. He was energized by the prospect of finally getting to do what he had always wanted. He made friends and had no trouble with the coursework, though spent many nights in the library studying and working on a neuroscience research project. During his second semester, he started dating a woman in his class. He kept in frequent phone contact with his mother, and her MS remained quiescent. His spirits were high.

Seven months prior to presenting to the clinic, around when his mother had an MS flare requiring a hospital admission, Jerome's anxiety worsened, and he began to worry about "almost everything." He ruminated about his mother's health, his grades, or whether his girlfriend would nag him for not spending enough time with her. His friends noticed he was more irritable, he had trouble focusing on textbook passages, and his thoughts kept him from falling asleep, leading to fatigue. He continued to socialize, having 3–4 drinks a day on weekend nights. Jerome noted that his exam grades went down "only slightly," but what he was really worried about was his clinical preceptorship on Monday mornings. Whenever he had to stand by a patient's bedside to present their case, he would become dizzy with intense anxiety that he would say something wrong, embarrassing, or inappropriate in front of the patient, preceptor, and other students. On one occasion, he had to excuse himself to sit down and sip a glass of water. He still received good feedback from his preceptor but was worried that he had come across as a "weak child" to his classmates. Furthermore, what would happen when he got to the "big league" of clerkships? The final straw came a week prior to coming to clinic, when he broke up with his girlfriend after an argument about him studying too much, ending the nine month relationship. This was all indicative of GAD in his eyes. Psychiatric review of systems was unremarkable. To Dr. Stone, Jerome appeared as a well-dressed young man, with a caduceus pin affixing his tie to his shirt. His mood was "not bad," with a reactive affect and orderly behavior. He frequently seemed to be searching Dr. Stone's face for approval.

Principles of Diagnosis and Management

Diagnosis

Assuming an accurate symptom inventory, the preferred diagnosis in this case is generalized anxiety disorder (GAD). The patient has had more than 6 months of socially and academically impairing worry, along with difficulty concentrating, irritability, early insomnia, and fatigue. This is on a background of being a moderately anxious person with high professional aims. However, the differential is important and includes adjustment disorder with anxious features, panic disorder, performance anxiety, and alcohol-induced anxiety disorder. Additionally, major depressive disorder and an unspecified personality disorder should be considered though are lower on the differential.

His anxiety symptoms appear to reach the level of a diagnosable disorder, though could be in line with the expected, normal anxiety from the trials of medical school. His intense anxiety with dizziness during bedside rounds might indicate panic attacks, though it seems to be on a spectrum of his everyday ruminative thoughts, and he denied other panic symptoms. His alcohol use on the weekends may be exacerbating or, less likely, primarily driving his anxiety on Monday mornings. Notably, his drinking may be culturally appropriate, to the degree that his peers are also binge drinking.

He described neurovegetative symptoms that could be part of a depressive syndrome, and his "irritability" could be a proxy for a depressed mood; nonetheless, he was denying depressed mood and anhedonia and did not have significant features of depression on exam.

Although the patient's childhood antecedents are presumably contributing to his presentation, at first glance he does not have a DSM-5 personality disorder, given healthy interpersonal relationships and a consolidated identity without severe behavioral disturbances.

Lastly, Jerome's case should certainly be considered in the context of the medical student experience. While he presents with an overt request to be given a diagnosis, his difficulties may not necessitate a diagnostic label and could alternatively be conceptualized as less than effective coping in response to stressors. If a diagnosis were needed in such a case, adjustment disorder with anxious features would be an apt reflection of the situation.

Management and Treatment

GAD is treated with medication and/or psychotherapy, often based on patient preference and profile. Typically, patients are treated with a serotonin reuptake inhibitor (SRI) medication; a benzodiazepine may be used cautiously and temporarily if acute relief is needed for the anxiety, physical tension, and insomnia. Many different types of therapy have a proven benefit for GAD, including cognitive behavioral therapy (CBT), psychodynamically oriented therapies, and "third-wave" treatments such as mindfulness-based stress reduction (MBSR). Alcohol use counseling and motivational interviewing would be beneficial if further exploration of his use revealed an alcohol-related disorder or if alcohol use was thought to be contributing to some of his symptoms.

More specifically to Jerome, based on preliminary history, he may benefit from a psychodynamically informed treatment, given the threads of separation difficulties, role confusion, loss, guilt, and perfectionism that run through his history.

From a coping and resilience point of view, Dr. Stone might choose, in articulating his formulation to Jerome, to describe his troubles as a response to a higher intensity of acute and chronic stressors than he is accustomed to, for which his usual coping mechanisms may not be fully adequate. Rather than speaking in terms of a disorder, such as GAD, and treating it through a "medical model" (i.e., assigning a diagnosis which is managed with a prescribed course of treatment), Dr. S could consider presenting to him an alternate framework – one in which Jerome might see himself as struggling with a real situation that would test even the most hardy individual and as having the agency to strengthen his coping strategies and enhance his resilience while learning tools that would serve him indefinitely over the lifetime of stressors that he will continue to face.

If medication is needed, an SRI would be the treatment of choice, having good tolerability and effectiveness in a wide variety of anxiety disorders. Further, an SRI would treat an undiagnosed depressive disorder and perhaps allow for some reduction of overly critical thoughts about self and related ruminations. Benzodiazepines should be used cautiously and with good risk counseling, as when anxiety is high and coping skills are being taxed, an individual may be at risk for escalating use; combining these medications with excess alcohol would also be a potential danger to review explicitly with the student.

Principles for Doctors Treating Doctors

Developed societies with rich economies that allow for longer periods of education have encouraged a trend toward an extended duration of adolescence, in which the student remains dependent on the family and their role is viewed as different from other adult occupations. Students run up against new academic demands in higher education, presenting threats to their precarious self-esteem [1]. Medical students are no exception. They must go through several costly years of undergraduate and medical school, often in addition to gap years for research, volunteering, or temporary employment. Once graduating, they are faced by the prospect of residency and specialization through fellowship training. Many are burdened by geographic displacements and must cut off nascent relationships at each stage. Bereft of money and forever occupied as a student, such a lifestyle may present barriers to becoming a full-fledged adult.

Therefore, it was unsurprising to Dr. Stone that Jerome, already at risk with his personal history, was struggling with anxiety and guilt around separating from his mother and forming lasting romantic relationships in a faraway city. During the second session, when discussing treatment options, Jerome adamantly refused medication because he did not want to rely on it. Despite reassurances for confidentiality, he also did not want to enter individual therapy; expressing irritation and discomfort at the prospect, he asked Dr. Stone if this would lead to him being "reported" to the school administration as a problem student.

During the initial engagement process, Dr. Stone recalled that Jerome's father was a Buddhist; Jerome had fondly recounted spending every Sunday with him meditating on the shore of a nearby lake. Jerome accepted Dr. Stone's suggestion for mindfulness-based stress reduction (MBSR) at a community center. He agreed that this sounded like a fairly good idea. He felt he could trust the treatment more if it were disconnected from the university, anticipated that it would be easier to tell his peers about it because it did not seem like traditional psychiatric treatment, and had a sense of wanting to reconnect with his experiences meditating. He agreed to follow up with Dr. Stone every two to four weeks, and over the next few months Jerome's anxiety improved, he focused better on schoolwork and on rounds, and he felt less irritable. He tentatively reconciled with his girlfriend but continued to struggle with intimacy. Through cultivation of mindfulness, he became aware of just how self-critical his thoughts were, even over small matters.

Generally, *mindfulness meditation* encompasses several practices and goals. It seeks to improve attention regulation through focus on various meditation objects so as to develop an improved capacity to be more fully in the present and take a non-judgmental stance toward one's self, thoughts, and feelings, as well as those of others. Some meditation practices, such as *vipassana, (Sanskrit: "insight")*, strive toward the development of a specific kind of insight about the transience of mental phenomena and the illusory nature of the self. The neuroscience literature suggests that various types of meditation can improve regulation of attention, emotion, and awareness [2]. MBSR and the closely related mindfulness-based cognitive therapy (MBCT) are part of what some call the "third wave" of CBT. MBSR was created by Dr. Jon Kabat-Zinn as a more standardized, clinically applicable method of implementing mindfulness meditation treatment [3]. It has proven efficacy in GAD [4] and has been shown to reduce employee stress [5].

Over subsequent sessions, after starting clinical rotations, Jerome would describe to Dr. Stone coming home drained, often experiencing his patients' suffering as his own. It was easy to empathize with them after having had firsthand experience with his mother. The critical voice in the back of his head became louder, often delivering a biting commentary about how he was failing his patients. He had yet to connect this with his childhood experience of needing to take care of his mother. Jerome added a loving-kindness meditation to his routine that he had learned in his course; he would repeat mantras with the intention for himself and others to be free of suffering and truly happy. Germer and Neff define self-compassion as having three parts: self-kindness, a sense of the universality of humanity, and de-identification with pain [6]. This has been applied clinically through compassion-focused therapy, which shows early potential, especially for those with high self-criticism or shame, or an avoidant style [7, 8]. Bloom argues that under many circumstances compassion is a healthier, more productive choice than empathy. "Unmitigated communions," or repeatedly putting oneself "into the shoes" of others (including patients), may lead to burnout. In contrast, to practice compassion means to be unilaterally kind, warm, and caring toward others, which does not require higher level cognitive or emotional empathy with the other. However, it would not be a stretch to say that an empathic connection remains vital for understanding patients and forming a strong alliance, especially in therapy [9]. Epstein's comparative analysis of Buddhism and psychoanalytic theory has attempted to reconcile the two and has convincingly responded to Rolland and Freud's objection to mindfulness meditation and religious practices as merely the pursuit of an "oceanic feeling" [10].

The demands and peculiarities of medical school may lead some students whose problems do not rise to a pathological level to seek psychiatric help. Selecting those who need psychiatric treatment may be challenging. One must not invalidate the student's struggles, such as by dismissing their concerns as part of a "medical student syndrome" (i.e. the partial identification with a diagnosis in the learning process) or otherwise leave them with an unfavorable experience that closes the door to future help-seeking. However, assigning a clinical diagnosis to a common response like normal anxiety around grades could over-prioritize adaptation to the patient role, and lead to regressive behavior or loss of resilience. Developing and sharing a conceptualization with the student about how stressors, coping skills, lifestyle behaviors, and personality factors may all be interacting to cause distressing or impairing symptoms are one way to offer the student a narrative for understanding the current situation and for setting the stage for further development of insight and curiosity about oneself. For students not needing clinical treatment, universal, wellness-type interventions sponsored by the school may be useful and have a low barrier to entry for those ambivalent about seeing a psychiatrist.

Finally, the transference and countertransference formed between the doctor and student-doctor as patient provide unique pitfalls and opportunities. In Jerome Ocean's case, Dr. Stone was able to understand his academic challenges from his own personal experience and could admire him for his dedication in caring for his mother, seeing this as a portent of a robust physicianly attitude. However, Dr. Stone also became aware of a fleeting, sadistic wish for his patient to go through the same "harsh" training process that he had as a student during a more demanding era in which the student's attention to their own emotional well-being was not a priority and even at times explicitly devalued. Such a countertransference would make it more difficult for the physician provider to empathize or offer validation to a student-patient with mild symptoms that present as "normal" responses to a situation (e.g., the "worried well" student). Awareness of such counter-transference responses, and understanding of the student-patient as an individual, rather than as a member of a broader group, will help the psychiatrist to develop a therapeutic approach to the patient. Reassurance and normalization can then be offered in a way that is validating and encourages further self-awareness for the student-patient, rather than in a manner that could be experienced as silencing or shaming. In other words, the message that "med school is tough, but if I made it, you can too!" can be conveyed spitefully or with compassion.

Outcome

With the boon of more self-compassion, Jerome's anxiety continued to improve. He grew closer to his girlfriend and found himself feeling less preoccupied with his mother's health.

While he still worried, he felt more able to come up with specific actions he could take to help her rather than an overwhelming sense of "powerlessness." During his clerkships, he cared for his patients without feeling inundated by their problems. Late in medical school, he worked with Dr. Stone in a brief psychodynamic treatment, offering an opportunity to explore his early life and his relationships with others – not things that were focused on in his mindfulness practices. He began to verbalize guilt he felt over not being able to help his mother enough and dug deeper into the psychological impact of his father's loss and having to take care of his mother as a child. He matched in neurology and completed a fellowship in multiple sclerosis at his home state's university hospital.

Pearls
- For medical students, the transition to adulthood is complicated by financial and time constraints, geographic displacements, and a prolonged identity as a student.
- Medical school confronts students with new academic demands and realities different from their idealized dreams. The typical stress and anxiety of medical school makes it more challenging to differentiate students needing psychiatric treatment from those who do not.
- Previously successful or healthy students can find it shaming and difficult to seek professional mental health treatment. Less traditional approaches to mental well-being may be less daunting there is mounting theoretical, neuroscientific, and clinical evidence for treatments such as MBSR/MBCT and compassion-focused therapy.
- The relationship between a doctor and student-doctor provides unique therapeutic value. So use it!

References

1. Elson M, editor. The Kohut seminars on self psychology and psychotherapy with adolescents and young adult. Ontario, Canada: Penguin Books Canada Ltd; 1987.
2. Tang YY, Hölzel BK, Posner MI. The neuroscience of mindfulness meditation. Nat Rev Neurosci. 2015;16(4):213–25.
3. Kabat-Zinn J. Full catastrophe living: using the wisdom of your body and mind to face stress, pain, and illness. New York: Bantam Books; 2013.
4. Hoge EA, Bui E, Marques L, et al. Randomized controlled trial of mindfulness meditation for generalized anxiety disorder: effects on anxiety and stress reactivity. J Clin Psychiatry. 2013;74(8):786–92.
5. Janssen M, Heerkens Y, Kuijer W, van der Heijden B, Engels J. Effects of mindfulness-based stress reduction on employees' mental health: a systematic review. PLoS One. 2018;13(1):e0191332.
6. Germer C, Neff K. Self-compassion in clinical practice. J Clin Psychol. 2013;69(8):856–67.
7. Leaviss J, Uttley L. Psychotherapeutic benefits of compassion-focused therapy: an early systematic review. Psychol Med. 2015;45(5):927–45.
8. Mackintosh K, Power K, Schwannauer M, Chan SWY. The relationships between self-compassion, attachment and interpersonal problems in clinical patients with mixed anxiety and depression and emotional distress. Mindfulness. 2018;9(3):961–71. https://doi.org/10.1007/s12671-017-0835-6.
9. Bloom P. Against empathy: the case for rational compassion. New York: HarperCollins Publishers; 2016.
10. Epstein M. Beyond the oceanic feeling: psychoanalytic study of Buddhist meditation. In: Molino A, editor. The couch and the tree: dialogues in psychoanalysis and Buddhism. New York: North Point Press; 1998.

Index

© Springer Nature Switzerland AG 2019
J. S. Gordon-Elliott, A. H. Rosen (eds.), *Early Career
Physician Mental Health and Wellness*,
https://doi.org/10.1007/978-3-030-10952-3